21ˢᵗ century medicine

A guide to bio-electronic regulatory techniques and complex
homoeopathy, systems which may provide us with the
medicine of the future.

With best wishes
Julian Kenyon
April 1986
Toronto.

By the same author:
CLINICAL ECOLOGY
    (with Dr G. T. Lewith)
MODERN TECHNIQUES OF ACUPUNCTURE
    Volumes 1, 2 and 3

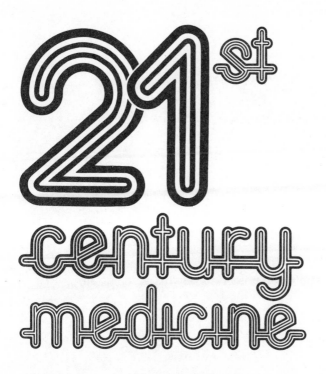

A Layman's Guide to the Medicine of the Future

by

Julian N. Kenyon
M.D., M.B., Ch.B.

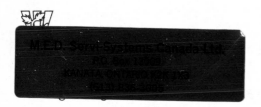

M.E.D. Servi-Systems Canada Ltd.
P.O. Box 13399
KANATA ONTARIO K2K 1X5
(613) 836-3886

First published 1986

Dedication

To Abigail and those unseen forces that guide us all.

British Library Cataloguing in Publication Data

Kenyon, Julian N.
   21st century medicine.
   1. Theraputic systems
   I. Title
   615.5   R733

   ISBN 0-7225-1198-1

Printed and bound in Great Britain

Contents

Preface

This book is a layman's guide to what may be a large part of medicine for the future, from both a practical and conceptual point of view. It has been written in response to many requests from patients and doctors alike, to whom I taught the techniques described in this book. All of these methods have been covered in detail in the three volumes of *Modern Techniques of Acupuncture*, [1] which because of their academic nature are only accessible to the health professional or the informed layman. Much of this book is a lay version of the *Modern Techniques of Acupuncture* series. I have deliberately kept references to a minimum so as not to interrupt the flow of ideas. My purpose has been to explain concepts and introduce new ideas rather than to prove anything in the scientific sense.

The new system of medicine which this book describes is an amalgam of ancient and modern ways of looking at the body. The techniques described are known as bio-energetic regulatory techniques, and all look at the body from an energetic (electrical) point of view. Ironically the scientific underpinning for much of bio-energetic regulatory medicine (BER medicine) comes from modern physics. In my view it is likely that conventional medicine will begin to adopt more of the ideas and systems described here, albeit possibly in a modified form.

I have been consistently surprised by how quickly changes are occurring in conventional medicine, and it is perfectly feasible that by the late 1990s everyday medicine may well be making use of the techniques and ideas described in this book. The great minds in medicine have all recognized that medicine is a constantly shifting body of knowledge. Notable amongst these was Sir William Osler, the famous surgeon, who used to tell students in his final lecture that his most important lesson had been reserved for the last: 'Half of what you have been taught here is untrue. The trouble is we do not know which half'. This is a very important lesson to learn, but I would suggest that some of what is written in this book may help you to decide.

Throughout the text I have used the terms complementary and alternative medicine interchangeably as umbrella terms for the various natural therapies.

I would like to thank Mrs Glenys Whittington for undertaking the task of typing the various drafts of the manuscript. I would also like to thank my many friends and colleagues, too numerous to mention, who have helped crystallize the ideas contained in this book.

JULIAN KENYON
Southampton, 1985.

Introduction

Much of this book is an ideas' book and some of the concepts I have explained may require re-reading in order to understand them fully. I have attempted to be fair to the achievements of modern medicine, although many will consider me not to have been. I describe what I feel will be the ideas that may well underpin the medicine of the future. In that these ideas are radically different from those underpinning conventional medicine of today, they may be difficult to understand or believe. I have attempted to provide, where possible, scientific corroboration for these concepts.

A number of chapters describe an already existing system of medicine which relies on these concepts — bio-electronic regulatory medicine (BER medicine). It is the development of this particular system of medicine which is the most likely possibility for the everyday medicine of the future.

Several chapters are devoted to complex homoeopathy, which is the key therapeutic system in BER medicine. There is also a chapter enabling the lay-person to treat everyday acute illness themselves, using complex homoeopathy.

I have finished with a chapter on holism and a speculative look at the future of medicine. I hope all who read this book may find at least some of the ideas stimulating and relevant.

1. Sociological Trends and their Relationship to Health Care

It seems appropriate in a book whose main thesis is the importance of the dynamic relatedness of all things, to look at sociological change in the Western world and its relationship to changes in medicine.

We live in a time when sociological change is more rapid than at any time since the Renaissance.[1] Christine McNulty's paper on 'What the Public Want and Think', given to the second annual conference of the British Holistic Medical Association in September 1984, makes interesting reading and bears looking at in detail. She draws on nearly twenty years' research experience into social trends in most Western countries. Trends, trend maps and value groups are the tools McNulty has used to look at sociological change.

Sociological Trends
There are two main trends in the Western world today. One is called the informality and autonomy trend, which briefly encompasses a desire for a less structured, rigid lifestyle and a move towards more freedom in all aspects of life. The second important trend is towards the equality of the sexes with a fresh approach to such tasks as child rearing and looking after a family. Values are also changing, with an emphasis on more subjective feminine values as opposed to the old masculine reductionist set of values. More and more people now see life as a system consisting of body, mind and spirit and reject the old view that the body is a machine which needs patching up occasionally.

As far as health is concerned, more than 70 per cent of the population are concerned about physical fitness and are doing something about it, such as jogging, swimming or eating a healthy diet low in fats and refined sugars. This contrasts markedly with the position on the same subject fifteen years ago. As a consequence there is an increasingly held belief that we can take more responsibility for our own health instead of subscribing to the older, more fatalistic, passive view of illness.

Social groups
Sociologists have identified three main groups in the population; the sustenance group, the outer directed group and the inner directed group. The sustenance group are mostly in the lower income brackets and are most concerned about survival. They will go to their doctors for reassurance so that they can feel safe and secure.

The outer directed group is concerned most with esteem, that of others and self-esteem. These are the leaders of business, and they are strongly motivated by the need to get ahead. Everything they do is directed to external norms. They believe in the objective, reductionist and quantitative world.

The inner directed group are mainly concerned about internal norms and individual growth. It is this group that is showing the greatest interest in complementary therapies and, significantly, is the fastest growing group of the population in all the Western countries studied. Thirty-three per cent of the population in the United Kingdom at the present time can be put into the inner directed group. The proportion of inner directed people is less in France than in the UK, and greatest in Holland. Germany has less inner directeds than any other European country. In the United States 30 per cent of the population are in the inner directed category.

The difference between the three groups is best illustrated by their responses to a particular problem, such as eating less. The sustenance group eats less because food is too expensive. The 'outer directeds' eat less because they want to look good. The 'inner directeds' eat less because they want to feel good.

The inner directed group used to be idealistic socialists, but have now largely switched their political allegiances from left to right. It is interesting to note that nothing in present day main stream politics fits the inner directed group, so a political vacuum is developing. My own educated guess is that this vacuum will be filled by the 'Green' parties, who are becoming increasingly active world-wide, although at the present time they appear insignificant from a political point of view.

Social Value Groups
The three main social groups can be sub-divided into seven value groups. These are self-explorers, social resistors, experimentalists,

conspicuous consumers, belongers, survivors and the aimless.

The self-explorers are the most inner directed group. They are growing at a steady rate and now account for 17 per cent of the population. Females slightly predominate in this group (51 per cent as opposed to 49 per cent). The average age of this group is thirty-seven.

Social resistors are also inner directed. They are predominantly male and middle aged. They are conservative with a large 'C' and tend to espouse causes. This group accounts for 13 per cent of the population of the United Kingdom at the present time, and is static.

Experimentalists tend to be young (below thirty) and want to experience things and tend to take risks. They represent 12 per cent of the UK population at the present time. Like the social resistors they are stable at the moment.

Conspicuous consumers are motivated by prestige and status; they want to get ahead. Women predominate in this group (male conspicuous consumers are sometimes given the name tag 'achievers'). This group represents 12 per cent of the UK population at the present time and is growing.

The belongers are people who want to fit in and conform. Survivors are mostly from the lower income group and tend to be middle aged to elderly. The aimless group is polarized between the young and the old and is declining. They tend to be resigned to things and include people who turn to drugs. A worrying trend in this group is the increasing proportion of young people in it, even though as a whole it is declining.

Attitudes to health

For the survivors health is somebody else's problem, and they take little responsibility for their own bodies. The conspicuous consumers want somebody else to take responsibility for their health also. As a group they are just beginning to turn to alternative medicine. Experimentalists will try anything, and would take the lead if they thought there was something in it for them. Generally speaking all groups except the inner directed ones (self explorers and social resistors), look on the body as a machine which needs patching up from time to time. The group most interested in complementary therapies are the self-explorers and they deserve looking at in greater detail.

Self-explorers and their approach to health

The most important facts about the self-explorer group is that they are growing steadily all over the Western world, and are opinion formers and opinion leaders. In other words what self-explorers think and do and say is of greater future significance than the same factors in any other group.

Of all groups the self-explorers are most people-orientated. They want service from people and not from machines. They want to take time with people and want people to take time with them and take an interest in them. They want a more people-orientated medicine in which they can take an active part. They are empathetic and tolerant and want to deal with small organizations. They also want more information about treatments and their possible side effects. This group consists of people who inform the public about their rights; they expose scandals and draw attention to social injustice. Above all they want freedom of choice in both goods and services. Freedom of choice in medical services is particularly important to them. It isn't surprising to find that the nucleus of the burgeoning numbers of self-help groups is formed by self-explorers. As a group they are more concerned about the quality of life as opposed to its length.

Most self-explorers are actively involved in healthy eating and/or a regular exercise programme. As consumers they want more honest information and distrust many of the platitudes of big business and big government. They want the ability to be creative and they are anti-authoritarian. They see conventional medicine, with its rigid inward-looking referal systems and hierarchical structures, as being authoritarian. As a result, because of many of the factors mentioned, they are turning to complementary therapies in large numbers. This trend is accelerating rapidly and it is only belatedly that the medical profession has begun to realize this, this realization being marked by such events as the working party on alternative medicine set up by the British Medical Association in 1984 and the inauguration of the British Holistic Medical Association in 1983. Similar events have been and are occurring in other countries.

As a group the self-explorers have low exposure to the television side of the media and high exposure to radio and the printed media such as newspapers.

Conspicuous consumers and experimentalists —
their approach to health
These groups are the next biggest group with a growing interest in complementary medicine. They tend to be pro-technology. They need to be told in appropriate terms why they should take more

of an interest in their bodies. They need something which appeals to their status and as complementary medicine is now becoming fashionable it is enjoying increasing support from these two groups.

Preventive medicine
The self-explorers, not surprisingly in view of their opinion leader status, show the greatest interest in this area. They form a lot of the articulate grass roots support for movements such as organic farming, Greenpeace and Friends of the Earth.

Attitudes to Medicalization of Birth and Death
Ivan Illich in his book *Medical Nemesis*[2] drew attention to the excessive medicalization of death. Birth has also been subjected to the same degree of medicalization, as seen by the strenuous efforts of the medical profession to force all mothers to have their babies in hospital. The attitudes of the various sociological groups to the medicalization of birth and death is interesting. The self-explorers would rather give birth and die at home. The experimentalists prefer to live fast and die young, perhaps in an accident, but if they survive long enough they wish to have the privilege of passing the last few hours of their lives in an intensive care unit. The conspicuous consumers prefer a high technology hospital birth with as many machines as possible connected up to them. In terminal illness they want everything possible done to prolong life, whether or not they continue life as a human vegetable.

Cultural Changes
The changes in medicine which this book describes are not occurring in isolation. The first part of this chapter has shown how social change is acting as a catalyst to the more general acceptance of alternative therapies and the holistic approach. Parallel changes are occurring in many other fields, notably the rise of the women's movement, the increasing unpopularity of nuclear power and nuclear weapons, and perhaps most importantly in the field of work and economics. James Robertson in his book *The Sane Alternative*[3] considers five scenarios for the economic future:

1 'Business as usual' — with solutions along orthodox lines.
2 'Disaster' — war, revolution, famine, pollution.
3 'Authoritarian Control' — either of the right or the left.
4 'Hyper-expansion' — rapid growth of the super scientific industry.

5   'SHE' — the sane, humane and ecological future.

It is the last alternative which is strongly favoured by the self-explorers. There is increasing evidence that small, self-sufficient and self-reliant businesses with a humane and ecologically acceptable face are flourishing in increasing numbers.[4] Barring a nuclear conflagration there is every reason to suppose that the 'small is beautiful' creed, beloved of Schumacher, may become the norm in all areas of our lives.

Conclusion: the Paradigm Shift

It is becoming more generally accepted that we are going through a major shift in consciousness, probably greater than that which occurred during the Renaissance. The main difference is that the Renaissance occurred over 300 years, whilst our current paradigm shift started in the mid 1960s and is likely to reach its peak at the turn of the century. Characteristically such changes follow an 'S' shaped curve. We entered the bottom of the curve in the mid 1960s and are now climbing steeply to the top which we should reach by the end of the century. I have attempted in this chapter to provide hard evidence that such a change is occurring rather than rely on emotive, but in some quarters fairly meaningless, phrases such as the 'coming of the new age' etc. The objective evidence that these changes are occurring is best summarized in Fritjof Capra's book *The Turning Point*[5] and Peter Schwartz and J. Ogilvy's book *The Emergent Paradigm.*[6] All of this evidence lends credibility and importance to the central theme of this book.

2. History

Conventional Medicine

Until the beginning of the nineteenth century all medical practice was broadly speaking traditional, and at that time the last great cultural change of the Renaissance began to introduce Cartesian scientific materialism into medicine, as well as many other areas of human endeavour. From then on medical practice was increasingly based on experiment, statistical studies and organization. Faith and belief, which had been and still are important features of traditional health systems, were largely swept aside and replaced by reasoning, logic and intellect. Inevitably the subjective aspects of illness were relegated to a very poor second place. Disease was increasingly looked at from a reductionist point of view, splitting it down into its component parts with the extreme having been reached in the twentieth century with, for example, research concentrating on changes at the sub-cellular level in order to search for clues to the cause and potential cure of malignancy.

The birth of the drug era at the beginning of this century with the discovery of aspirin, cast the die for the direction conventional medicine was to follow, and with it the eternal search for Ehrlich's 'Magic Bullet'. Generally speaking a symptom suppression approach has been adopted by all areas of conventional medicine. The drug industry has somehow managed to hypnotize the doctors as well as the public.

The strides made by modern medicine must, however, be acknowledged, but with honesty, admitting that much of our increased longevity and reduction in the incidence of infectious disease has been due to public health measures and rising living standards and not to advances in medical science. Sadly we are not able to make the same claims as far as chronic disease is concerned. Modern medicine has produced a powerful and eminently successful approach to acute illness and to that extent it is unlikely to be bettered. A reductionist's approach to acute illness is eminently successful and appropriate. For example, it is pointless asking a patient with a broken leg if he is happy in his job or whether he eats healthy food. This is irrelevant to the acute situation. He needs his fracture setting. It is in the area of chronic illness that modern medicine has been unable to deliver the goods, and it has largely itself to blame for its reductionist suppressive approach.

Since the beginning of our present paradigm shift in the mid 1960s conventional medicine has found itself increasingly under fire. A notable landmark in the public reaction to drug based, high technology medicine was Ivan Illich's hard hitting book *Medical Nemesis*, published in 1975, with its main thesis being that doctors are a danger to health. He drew on an impressive range of evidence, including the embarrassing finding that when doctors went on strike in Bogota the mortality rate dropped significantly, only to go up again when they returned to work!

Slowly, and in the public's eyes belatedly, the medical profession has responded by showing an increasing interest in complementary therapies. The most important landmarks to date have been the establishment of the American Holistic Medical Association in 1978, and the British Holistic Medical Association in 1983.

Traditional Therapies
Most complementary therapies have arisen out of traditional therapies or are continuations of them. A good example is acupuncture which has survived virtually unchanged from its origins in China some 2,500 years ago. Osteopathy and chiropractic have developed from the old practice of bone setting. Herbal medicine has remained largely unchanged. The vast majority of practitioners in all disciplines of complementary medicine were non-medical up until the 1970s, when increasing numbers of doctors began to practice these therapies, most commonly acupuncture.

The value of traditional therapies were first officially recognized by the World Health Organization in 1976, which set up a traditional medicine section. They realized that 80 per cent of the world's population, particularly those living in rural areas, made exclusive use of traditional practitioners for their medical needs. Interestingly enough some doctors looked on the discovery of well-organized systems of traditional practitioners in every country as providing a framework for the promulgation of conventional therapy and diagnostic techniques. Thankfully most traditional practitioners would not accept this, and the view that these practitioners should be recognized and respected in their own right was adopted by the World Health Organization.

The Rise of Acupuncture

In my view the rise of interest in acupuncture by the medical profession has been a fascinating phenomenon. Unlike many complementary therapies acupuncture works quickly, particularly in relieving pain, and is somehow reminiscent of the action of a drug. It therefore holds a lot of appeal for doctors and patients alike as it can be seen to work, often within minutes. The discovery that a mechanism may be at work causing the body to release a natural pain-killer called endorphin, was, and is, largely responsible for the continued and increasing medical interest in this treatment. Doctors were shown a mechanism identical to that of a drug to explain why acupuncture worked. This appealed to the drug based 'mind-set' of conventional medicine and consequently interest has grown rapidly. In my view this tells us more about how the medical mind thinks than how acupuncture works.

The net result of all of this has been many papers on the subject of acupuncture, sufficient even to satisfy the most conservative medical journals that there is convincing evidence that it works.

From the classical point of view acupuncture can be placed, albeit rather forcefully and wrongly in my view, in the western neuro-physiological mould. This has been an advantage from the point of view of increasing medical interest in alternative therapies but a disadvantage from the point of view of research into what the traditional acupuncturist considers its mechanism of action to be.

Interest in other alternative therapies has largely sprung from an introduction to this area of medicine via acupuncture. Very slowly a small number of doctors are beginning to see the broader implications of acupuncture in particular and alternative medicine in general, and these will be discussed more fully in the following chapter.

Homoeopathy

Homoeopathy owes its origin to a German physician, Samuel Hahnemann, working in the latter half of the eighteenth century. Briefly, he realized the principle of treating an illness with an infinitesimal dose of a substance which, when given in its concentrated form, would produce the same symptoms as shown by the patient being treated. The correct remedy to give is called the similimum, and the art of homoeopathy largely depends upon matching the patient's clinical picture to a drug picture. This approach to homoeopathy is the classical one, and has tended to be followed in a somewhat doctrinaire fashion, possibly encouraged by the fact that homoeopathy was shunned by conventional medicine, and as a result the homoeopathic doctors tended to form somewhat inward looking medical societies. Classical homoeopathy[1] has remained largely unchanged since Hahnemann's day.

Complex homoeopathy

Towards the end of Hahnemann's life a number of prominent homoeopaths started giving more than one remedy at the same time (anathema to the classical homoeopath). This practice was vigorously suppressed by the other homoeopaths who would not countenance such a contravention of classical homoeopathic dogma. Consequently a rigid approach to homoeopathy became the norm, and has tended to remain so to the present day, with the result that homoeopathy has, in comparison with other medical disciplines, stood still for the past 150 years. The German homoeopaths, however, did develop the idea of giving multiple remedies, as they perceived that patients required more than one remedy at the same time. This was most often the case in chronic illness. Acute self-limiting illness could, and still can, be effectively treated with classical single remedy homoeopathy.

Towards the end of the nineteenth century the mixing of remedies became more sophisticated and was based upon empirical observation. The aim was to produce compatible mixtures with a broad range of action (it is well known amongst homoeopaths that some remedies do not mix well with others and are therefore incompatible). Soon herbal remedies were added to these mixtures, so adding all the advantages of traditional herbal medical practice to the knowledge of the classical homoeopath. The main advantages of herbal medicine are the use of drainage remedies (to increase elimination via the colon, kidney and skin), and lymphatic remedies etc. The net result was a therapeutic system called complex homoeopathy which combined herbal and low potency homoeopathic remedies. The mixtures were specific for particular indications, had a broad scope of action and were easy to use. Slowly the complex homoeopathic system has taken over from classical homoeopathy in Germany where it now accounts for approximately 80 per cent of all homoeopathy practised. Curiously this revolution in homoeopathy has been largely restricted to Germany and has only recently spread to other countries. Complex homoeopathy is the most important and widely used therapeutic system in the techniques described in this book, and will be discussed in depth in Chapter 8.

Specialization in Alternative Medicine

The tradition of specializing in medicine has, curiously enough, been carried over into complementary medicine. Perhaps this is something to do with the inordinate respect which our society gives to the specialist. Therefore the norm has been to become an osteopath, acupuncturist or homoeopath. It is only since the early 1980s that doctors have realized that a number of skills are necessary in order to sort out most problems, and a new breed of doctor has begun to appear, one with skills in a number of disciplines. This doctor is one who is generalist in approach but specialist in capability. This in my view should be the hallmark of the doctor of the future.

Conclusion

The rift between natural medicine and conventional medicine, which has increased ever since it began some 180 years ago, now seems to be healing. We now have the exciting possibility that the future evolution of conventional scientific medicine will be largely shaped by the ideas underpinning alternative medicine. In my view this will ultimately lead to a truly scientific and causally directed system of medicine, with all the manifold benefits that this implies.

3. Concepts in Medicine

The systems of medicine described in this book are called bio-electronic regulatory techniques (BER). They all look at various electrical parameters as being indicative of organ function and pathology (organ damage) in the body. The ideas behind these methods have come from various disciplines within alternative medicine, particularly acupuncture, all of which have some concept of energy flow in the body. These techniques build upon the already solid scientific base of conventional medicine to form an altogether more advanced system of medicine. However, the concepts underlying bio-electronic regulatory medicine are very different to those underpinning conventional medicine. In order to understand this important point it is necessary to look at concepts in science, particularly physics, and their relationship to bio-energetic regulatory medicine.

Conventional medicine has a mechanistic and somewhat static view of the body. This is well illustrated by looking at the investigative methods of conventional medicine which use X-ray technology and other body scanning techniques to look at the body. These are able to visualize structure in the body in remarkable detail, particularly with the use of the recently developed nuclear magnetic resonance techniques. Unfortunately looking at structure alone, no matter how detailed, is of limited value as it tells us nothing about function. It therefore doesn't give us any signposts as to whether disordered function is present, which may ultimately lead to structural pathological change. From the point of view of treatment this is an important consideration as it is often too late to be able to do something effective when disease has reached this relatively late stage. In conceptual terms conventional scanning techniques are a reflection of the current mechanistic scientific model.

Concepts in Science and Their Relevance to Medicine

To understand the inadequacy of current concepts it is necessary to look at the revolution in thought which took place in physics at the beginning of this century. The old classical (Newtonian) mechanistic view of the world with independent building blocks gave way to concepts of pattern, process and interrelatedness. These concepts are fundamental to our most accurate description of reality as contained in the discipline of modern physics. This points to a unified as opposed to a fragmented world view. David Bohm in his book *Wholeness and the Implicate Order*[1] points out that a mechanistic world view as consisting of separate entities, one affecting the other but not producing any change in the essential nature of each entity as a result of interaction, is no longer tenable. He goes on to state that modern physics points to relationships and interactions in which the parts are themselves changed somehow as a result of interacting, one with another. Bohm concludes that this sort of interaction is more reminiscent of the interconnectedness of a biological system than that of a mechanistic system such as a clock. It is interesting how closely this view corresponds to that of the ancient Chinese philosophers. Acupuncture, for example, is seen by Manfred Porkert[2] in his book *The Theoretical Foundation of Chinese Medicine: Systems of Correspondence*, as being essentially a system of relationships, with the relationships themselves being of greater practical importance than the parts to which they refer. In this way acupuncture, by means of the various meridians and their connections, relates the elbow to particular points on the arm, to the knee on the same side, to the elbow on the opposite side and to a point on the ear. This therefore gives a number of ways of treating the elbow, and is in many ways more useful than knowing everything about the elbow itself.

Modern medicine continues to have a fragmented, uncoordinated approach, not least in the way it is constituted into separate specialities. This situation is compounded by the various private health insurance schemes who only see specialist treatment as worthy of recognition. Any general approach is, by implication, second-class. To the critical observer specialism in medicine leads to vested interest, a narrow view and, in some cases, tragically inappropriate therapy. Ironically, as pointed out previously, the specialist approach has been carried over into alternative medicine where it is the norm to become an acupuncturist, a homoeopath or an osteopath, etc. and again just as in mainstream medicine, vested interest and a narrow view all too often appear.

Conceptual Differences Between Mainstream and Alternative Medicine

If the conceptual differences between mainstream and alternative medicine came to be generally understood, then innovative research projects would become more commonplace and a healthy trend away from specialization would perhaps appear. These conceptual differences find expression in the concept of biological energy common to most forms of alternative medicine, and also the holistic approach integral to most disciplines within alternative medicine. Because alternative therapies in general and bio-energetic regulatory medicine in particular are couched in terms of biological energy, they tend to have an intrinsically dynamic view of the body with concepts such as energy flow, change in the patient's condition, etc. being everyday ideas used to understand all clinical situations. The idea of biological energy is developed to a greater or lesser degree in different therapies, but probably finds its most sophisticated expression in traditional Chinese medicine (acupuncture) where this energy is termed chi. The flow of chi along the superficial and deep branches of the various meridians is the key to understanding the relationships (known as causal chains) shown by bio-energetic regulatory techniques (see Chapter 5). The idea of biological energy is developed in a slightly different way, but perhaps in as sophisticated a sense in homoeopathy: the energetic, flowing, changing view of the body necessitates a connected and therefore holistic view of the patient's problem. In other words, all aspects of the problem are seen in terms of their relatedness to each other, just as in the world view seen by modern physics. It comes as something of a surprise to realize that conventional medicine is the only medical system ever known to man which has no concept of biological energy. This is one of its major differences to alternative medical approaches, the other important difference is its fragmented narrow view.

Research Trends in Alternative Medicine

The current bio-medical model is dominated by the Cartesian approach, with its separation of the mind and body and concentration on individual parts. The implication is that advances will come from concentrating on ever smaller parts of the human automaton, evidenced by the current emphasis on molecular biology. Nevertheless, molecular biology has been and continues to be spectacularly successful, probably too much so as this has produced a reductionist *ad absurdam* approach to medical research. As a result we have lost our ability to see things in context and to recognize the importance of relationships. The generalist approach is losing out to the more prestigious specialist (and narrow) approach. Most important of all is the neglect of the mind and its effect on the physical. This will be dealt with in detail in Chapter 6.

Ironically, Descartes, even though he was responsible for the mind/body split, did emphasize the importance of the connections between the two. Like all great thinkers he saw the limitations of his mind/body split; our narrow interpretation of this approach is our responsibility and not Descartes'. The net result is difficulty in raising support for innovative research couched in the bio-energetic paradigm.

A change in our bio-medical model is therefore long overdue, but to be effective this must start at the top with the research committees who have control on research funding. At the time of writing the future looks bleak from this point of view.

Research into alternative medicine is best illustrated by looking at acupuncture research. It is striking that the main approach to acupuncture is from the nervous system and biochemical point of view, the psychological approach coming a poor third. An energetic approach looking at subtle electrical change hardly figures at all and is clearly regarded as a non-starter at best by the scientific community. Yet the fact remains that acupuncture was conceived by the Chinese entirely in terms of energy flow in the body and these ideas form the corner-stone of bio-energetic regulatory medicine. The main reason for the present direction of research into acupuncture is due to the conflict of concepts discussed earlier. It may be that one important reason for this is that research paradigms for nervous system and biochemical research already exist, therefore any investigation couched in these terms is easy to set up and so appears inherently more reasonable. Research paradigms which involve an energetic approach are not well developed, and are consequently difficult to fund. As a result these approaches often appear 'wrong-headed'. This is of major importance in holding back scientific progress in the area of bio-energetic regulatory medicine. Key areas of research in this area will have to struggle through in order that these new approaches establish a real foothold within scientific medicine. This important question is dealt with in detail in the final chapter of this book.

It would be wrong to think that research directed at nervous system and biochemical questions isn't valuable. On the contrary, these approaches will produce mountains of 'good research' which will be published in respectable journals but it may not in the long run produce anything worth knowing. The outlook for more innovative approaches geared to looking at the energetic aspects of acupuncture is gloomy, as it is not feasible that such ideas would receive sufficient support from research bodies as their funds are largely controlled by conventional doctors who appear less likely to back these new initiatives.

The Theory of Dissipative Structures

Looking at the body using BER techniques shows that nobody is ever 100 per cent healthy. It is of considerable importance to try and find some validation for this curious result, otherwise these methods could be interpreted as registering random meaningless fluctuations only, or it could be said that they are so prone to error due to the technology used that this error must constitute most of what is being recorded. However, the work of the brilliant Belgian chemist Ilya Prigogine[3] lends support to the veracity and relevance of BER techniques.

Prigogine was awarded the Nobel Prize in 1977 for his theory of dissipative structures. Briefly, the classical view of the universe is that it has a tendency to entropy, in other words it is slowly running down. In contrast, biological systems display an opposite tendency, thereby contradicting Newton's second law of thermodynamics (i.e. a glass of hot water, if left, will cool down until it reaches the energy level [temperature] of its environment). Prigogine describes, through a series of complex mathematical equations, how the second law can remain valid for the universe as a whole, but will fail when applied to certain parts, particularly biological systems. Prigogine calls such structures dissipative structures, implying that they interact with their local environment by consuming energy from it. A fundamental feature of these structures is that the greater the energy flow required to maintain them, the greater the susceptibility to disruption, due to outside change. This quality of fragility is paradoxically the key to growth. By responding in a coherent way to this perturbation the dissipative structure (i.e. the body) is able to escape to a higher level of complexity, as a result of successfully coping with the disruption. In other words the disruption is essential in order to allow for further growth by means of a consequent re-ordering of the dissipative structure.

This theory must have implications for biology in general and for medicine in particular. The implications are interesting for two reasons. First, they assign a fundamental biological role to illness. In other words illness, and indeed various levels of continuing illness, are essential in order for any dissipative structure to survive and develop. Secondly, the idea of producing solutions from outside the body in terms of suppressive drugs or, in some cases, surgery appears wrong-headed when considered alongside Prigogine's theory. These solutions do not produce any fundamental reordering in the body. On the other hand, therapies which help the body in its effort to reorganize to higher levels of complexity (i.e. to recover from illness), by stimulating the body to react positively to disruption, appear the only tenable form of medicine in terms of this theory. Prigogine's work therefore provides an important theoretical backing for bio-electronic regulatory medicine and for causally directed stimulatory therapeutic approaches which are the core of the new system of medicine described in this book. Any approach which depresses the body's capacity to react positively to treatment (which is what most supressive therapy does) is going to be counter-productive. This is a central criticism of conventional approaches and will be dealt with in more detail in the next chapter.

Conclusion

In order to reach a balanced view it is important to recognize that a number of major advances have come from looking at the body in ever smaller parts, right down to the molecular level. This is the reductionist approach *par excellence*, and to deny its success would be dishonest. There is a natural tendency to react against scientific reductionism in an extreme manner, with the danger of throwing out the baby with the bath water. The end in view should be a system of medicine the concepts of which are balanced between reductionism and holism. Bio-energetic regulatory medicine is just such an approach. For example, it wouldn't attempt to treat a problem where the fundamental cause was abnormal bacteria in the bowel by recommending a vague stress reduction approach. It would replace the missing normal bacteria and get rid of the abnormal ones, which is essentially a reductionist approach but entirely in keeping with the natural tendency of the body.

I have perhaps over-stated the cause for quantum physics, so to redress the balance it is important to understand that Newtonian physics is still applicable to all large scale systems. The physics of biological systems are probably different in that they appear to require a reductionist mechanistic Newtonian approach in some aspects and a holistic quantum physical approach in others. The net result should be a balance between the two.

4. Causally Directed Therapy Versus Symptom Suppression

Everyone, including the medical profession, would readily agree that treating the cause is the best way of coping with any illness. Clearly we live in a world in which the law of cause and effect operates in all things. However, in practice conventional medicine often pays lip service only to the idea of causal treatment whilst it mostly indulges in gross suppressive therapy for the majority of chronic diseases, and many acute ones as well.

Chronic Illness
The symptom suppression approach is well illustrated by looking in detail at the way in which a specific chronic illness is treated by conventional medicine. Rheumatoid arthritis is a good choice as it is relatively common and usually proves difficult to treat, both from a conventional and an alternative point of view. The average rheumatoid patient has a wide battery of blood tests and X-ray investigations when being looked at in a conventional manner. These all delimit in a highly sophisticated way a number of abnormalities in the immune system and the level of damage in various joints. The vast majority of investigations delineate the state of the disease at that time. Very few investigations are carried out with the view to asking the question 'What caused this patient's problem?' In fact the majority of them have no relevance at all to this question. Modern medicine is very good at 'throwing the book' at the patient, and many times the patient is investigated to death, in some cases literally (certain investigations such as carotid angiography, a technique used to visualize the blood vessels in the head, carries a significant mortality rate). Some authorities, effectively silenced by their conventional counterparts, claim that X-rays themselves are dangerous (although in fairness conventional medicine recognizes that X-ray examination should be avoided in pregnancy).

When it comes to treatment the story is totally different. The sufferer with rheumatoid arthritis basically has a choice of four different approaches, all suppressive and often used in combination. They are pain-killers, anti-inflammatory drugs, steroids (these powerfully suppress the body's natural inflammatory response) and immune system suppressants. The patient may well wonder what is the point of all the sophisticated and expensive investigation if he is going to end up on the same treatment as all other rheumatoids. In other words there appears to be little relationship between the sophistication of the investigations and the subsequent treatment, and there would probably be no significant difference in the patient's condition if they were treated conventionally with one or a combination of the previously mentioned therapies after having undergone a clinical diagnosis and only one blood test at the most! The money saved by the hospital service by using this simpler approach (and in the end effectively getting the same clinical result) would account for a sizeable sum!

The conclusion is that medical science has accumulated vast amounts of information about specific conditions, mostly of a descriptive nature. This knowledge remains valid and useful but unfortunately hasn't altered the fundamental approach of conventional medicine to chronic disease. The very suggestion that rheumatoid arthritis could perhaps be cured and the destructive joint changes be made good is received with extraordinary vehemence by rheumatologists. It's almost as if they are threatened by any approach which might cure the problem. Sadly, this is typical of the pervasive therapeutic nihilism which seems to have invaded much of modern medicine, certainly as far as chronic illness is concerned.

Consequently, the chronically ill patient is placed in the worse possible environment in order to affect a cure. The patient's medical attendants pour scorn on any method which claims to contribute to a cure, so it is hardly surprising that the doctors' hopeless attitude to chronic disease is soon picked up and copied by the patient. If nothing else I hope my book will stimulate some anger amongst sufferers from chronic illness so that they can effectively criticize their doctors' approach to their problem and have the courage to stand up and do something about their illness, without being intimidated or threatened by withdrawal of medical care if they take their salvation into their own hands. There are signs that this healthy trend is beginning and that doctors with a proprietorial attitude to their patients will find it increasingly difficult to hold a viable practice together, especially as there is currently an abundance of doctors, which can only be good as far as the patients are concerned.

In contrast, the alternative approach to chronic illness invariably portrays an over-optimistic face, and in practice is never quite as successful as its public image would lead one to believe. However, it is to be hoped that this optimistic view of the results from treatment remains as this in itself increases the patient's motivation enormously and in the end means more successful therapy. However, this does not mean that we should not continue to try to establish, in an objective manner, the effectiveness or otherwise of various alternative treatments.

Acute Disease

The tendency of the medical profession to use a steam hammer to crack a nut is nowhere seen more clearly than in the indiscriminate use of antibiotics. Acute infections are very common indeed and have always been so. The current impression is that before the days of antibiotics then most of these patients would have succumbed, although, in fact, this is far from the truth. Before the days of antibiotics simple measures such as bed rest, increased fluid intake and various other techniques beloved and still used by naturopaths and enlightened doctors, were used in order to help the body's natural healing processes work to overcome the infection. Many homoeopaths argue that most infections are from bacteria which are normally present in the body anyway, such as Eschericia Coli which normally inhabits the bowel and is essential for all sorts of body functions. They ask the question: why do the body's own bacteria become pathogenic and grow in large numbers in certain instances? Some claim that the terrain of the body is the key; in other words in acute infection something happens to the body to allow the bacteria to become pathogenic and grow in excessive numbers. Even the venerable Louis Pasteur acknowledged this on his death bed with the statement that Claud Bernard (who realized the importance of the terrain) was right. Pasteur's famous words were 'the terrain is everything, the bacteria nothing'. It is important to realize that for Pasteur, who discovered the existence of bacteria, this statement was a complete volte-face.

In practice antibiotics ought to be reserved for the very few cases in whom infection becomes life threatening. An informed use of natural therapeutics and a healthy diet would reduce the number of such cases to an absolute minimum.

The indiscriminate use of antibiotics as a first line of treatment in infectious illness (much of it viral in origin anyway, against which antibiotics are useless) is one of many examples of inappropriate therapy which acts as a major cause of chronic disease. It does this by suppressing the body's natural defences and reactions, and thereby reduces their ability to correct the problem which originally caused the infection to appear. This idea is difficult for doctors to accept as it implies that much of their management of acute illness is not only useless but actually harmful, but the idea that the same applies to chronic illness as well gives much more cause for worry. Encouraging a natural resolution of underlying causes is a corner-stone of bio-electronic regulatory medicine and is the antithesis of conventional suppressive approaches.

Academic Respectability
The drug industry depends crucially on a sort of mass hypnosis for the continued success of its most profitable products. This effect has spread amongst the medical profession with whom it almost certainly started. The American Medical Association began the process by teaming up with the then infant drug industry and advertising its products. Of incidental interest is the fact that one of the reasons for setting up the AMA was to stamp out homoeopathy. Unbelievably enough at that time homoeopathy and herbal medicine seemed set to take over and dominate the American medical scene.[1]

The drug industry has provided considerable funds for medical research and as a result drug-based medicine has acquired the cloak of academic respectability. Review papers on, for example, the medical management of migraine or asthma are commonplace in medical journals. They amount to long lists of drugs, often referred to by their chemical names (somehow implying that this makes the whole thing more acceptable), which are at the same intellectual level as a cook discussing recipes for a casserole.

Is suppressive drug therapy harmful?
Neville Hodgkinson, in his book *Will to Be Well, The Real Alternative medicine*[2] claims that it is in the nature of conventional drug therapy to cause illness by suppressing symptoms for short term gain at the expense of weakening the patient in the long run. So a condition which might otherwise resolve naturally, once the initial flare-up of symptoms has passed, becomes chronically and progressively damaging instead. He gives the example of arthritis.

As joints are used, damage occurs. There is constant wear, which has to be made good. Cells have to be renewed and debris carried away in the blood. Arthritis pain occurs when this repair process is not taking place fast enough to keep up with the damage caused. Pain and inflammation help to reduce movement so that healing and waste disposal can catch up with the rate at which the damage is inflicted.

Drugs taken for the condition not only suppress the protective function of pain, but interfere at several different points with the repair system by which extra blood (and healing agents which the blood carries) is sent to the body sites needing repair. Most of these drugs also damage the stomach, allowing half digested substances to be absorbed into the blood stream thereby increasing the burden of the circulatory waste–disposal system.

So, it should be no surprise that with thousands of tons of anti-arthritic drugs being consumed every year, far from being conquered by the pharmaceutical 'emperor' this disease has become worse over the past 40 years and is one of the most prevalent in the west.

Another massive market is that for anti-hypertensives — drugs to lower blood pressure. Sometimes blood-pressure can go through the roof in a life threatening way, and there is then a strong case for emergency intervention with a pill. But the really big sales lie among the millions whose pressure is not out of control, but which has risen above the mean to levels associated with increased risk of heart trouble, or a stroke.

This association is treated as a cause but in fact, blood-pressure varies widely not only from minute to minute but from day to day and sometimes from month to month; and the changes are part of broad patterns of bodily adaption co-ordinated through the brain, in response to life's demands.

When someone goes through a particularly demanding period, blood-pressure may stay high as a part of a generalised increase in arousal, geared to resolving the difficulties. In such circumstances, to lower the blood-pressure with a drug may be the last thing a patient needs. By reducing blood flow and thereby interfering with the ability to cope at 'high pressure' medical treatment may ensure that the problems remain unresolved. Thus the condition becomes a chronic one.

Hodgkinson's last point is reminiscent of Prigogine's ideas which were discussed in Chapter 3. Hodgkinson's comment on the identification of the causes of illness and their treatment is as follows:

Doctors, blinkered by our society's materialistic outlook, have increasingly lacked insight into the real causes of illness and have used the thin veil spun by the pharmaceutical industry to cover up their own nakedness. We as patients have subscribed to the illusion only too readily, preferring to think that all our physical ailments are in some way separate to ourselves and therefore treatable by external agents, rather than to face the fact that it is our own troubled thoughts, feelings and actions that create the fertile bodily territory where illness can enter and flourish.

A balanced view

In spite of all the vehement criticism of the drug industry, their products are very powerful and they do work. In some situations they are essential and life saving. Asthma provides a good example. During the past few years a number of papers have appeared in medical journals concerning death due to asthma. They all clearly point to the conclusion that steriod therapy was introduced too late in those cases who succumbed, and the lives of most of them would have been saved if these drugs had been used early enough in high enough doses. Therefore a balanced view is necessary, as yet again we are in danger of throwing the baby out with the bath water.

Science and its Relevance to the Assessment of Therapy

Modern medical science demands proof before any therapy is accepted. This is part of the game and deception of science. Hodgkinson makes an interesting point on the assessment of the success of anti-hypertensive drugs. He mentions a research project conducted in Newcastle upon Tyne and published in the journal of The Royal College of General Practitioners in 1982. Seventy-five patients who had diastolic blood-pressures above 100 were treated and they were all questioned about their progress. The group consisted of 41 women and 34 men with an average age of 50. The doctors and a relative of each patient (a most unusual step in medical research) completed questionnaires. The doctors registered 100 per cent improvement. As far as they were concerned the drug had done its job of bringing the blood-pressure down. There had been no obvious side-effects and no complaints from the patients about the pills (the pills were mainly sympathetic blockers, diuretics and a commonly used anti-hypertensive drug). Nearly half the patients said they felt better (26 of the women and 10 of the men).

But when it came to the relatives, who might be expected to be the most objective in their assessment according to Hodgkinson, 74 out of the 75 judged the patients to have deteriorated on the drugs. Their memory, mood, initiative, energy and activity had declined, sometimes severely, and they were more anxious and irritable. In other words, it depends on which aspect of the therapy you care to investigate as to whether the proof is forthcoming.

Scientific assessment of diets

Natural therapy practitioners uniformly advise a low-fat, low-sugar diet and an avoidance of all chemical contaminants, such as food additives. Modern medicine demands conclusive proof of these measures before they can be adopted. A recent leading article in the British Medical Journal discussing diet and cancer concluded that there was some evidence that a low-fat diet lowers the incidence of this disease, but this was not yet proven in a manner acceptable to the medical profession. In this situation it is important to ask whether it is provable at all? The experiment required is almost too enormous to mount.

How good is science at assessing risks from chemicals?

Food additives give a useful insight into the validity of scientific investigation into toxic hazards. The accepted position is that they are safe. However, we do know that they accumulate in the body tissues to the extent that the corpses of habitual junk food eaters take longer to deteriorate! The immediate thought is that these chemicals must be harmful. But that isn't good enough, we need proof! It is important to examine the validity of the methods used by scientists to determine the toxicity of these chemicals, if we are to have any confidence in the official line that they are safe. Food additive toxicology relies on three sets of data to determine what is and is not safe. First, human epidemiology is looked at, but in relation to food additives this science is almost entirely useless. For example, cigarette smoking kills about 25 per cent of life-time smokers, but it took epidemiologists twenty-five years to demonstrate this fact in a scientifically acceptable manner. With some 3,500 or more food additives used in some thousands of products and in millions of combinations, in small quantities (in some cases using up to thirty different additives in a single product) then it becomes impossible for epidemiology to identify any long term or chronic effects of the use of particular food additives. In recent years a range of tissue culture tests have been devised. These so called short-term tests can identify some cancer-producing effects in test organisms. But at most these tests will detect only a specific sub-set of cancer causing chemicals; they are irrelevant to all other toxic hazards.

The regulation of food additives is based almost entirely upon animal tests. Only recently has there been any attempt to establish a quantitative estimate of the correlation between toxicity tests with laboratory animals and human toxicology for chemicals that are believed to cause cancer. This analysis, carried out by David Salsburg of Pfizer Central Research in America suggests that the animal tests are successful in identifying carcinogens (cancer-producing chemicals) only some 30 per cent of the time. This means that the results of the tests are wrong more often than they are right.

Not surprisingly, the Director of the British Industrial Biological Research Association points out that food additive toxicology is not a science which seeks to understand the biological effects of chemicals upon humans, but merely a technology designed to produce animal test data sufficient to gain permission from governments for the use of additives. There is disturbing evidence in view of a number of recent scandals concerning certain anti-arthritic drugs that the same applies to at least part of the drug industry.

It is important to ask whether the god of science makes us waste vast amounts of money and brain power attempting to prove things which are obvious anyway, or are ultimately unprovable. The sensible person accepts that chemicals are toxic and should be avoided and that a low-fat diet will lead to a longer and healthier life. The sceptic continues to eat these substances as the hazards are not proven and runs the risk, indeed the strong possibility, of succumbing to a chronic illness of one sort or another.

Reactive Capability
In order for the body to respond positively to a natural therapeutic approach it must be able to react. If its reactive capability is depressed for whatever reason, then the ability to get better is severely compromised. The main causes of poor reactive capacity are poor nutrition (particularly deficiency in micro-nutrients, such as vitamins and minerals), suppressive drug therapy, and severe illness of any sort. The first two causes are potentially avoidable. The effects of steroids on the body's reactive capacities are shown by the following *Segmental Electrogram* recordings. Normally following electrical stimulation the deflections of the recording widen, indicating some reaction of the body to the stimulation. Both these recordings are from patients who had been on steroids, one patient with asthma, the other with rheumatoid arthritis. Both recordings (Figures 1 and 2) are taken after electrical stimulation

and both show a virtually straight line recording. This contrasts with a typical recording of someone with normal reactive capacity shown before stimulation in Figure 3 and after stimulation in Figure 4. (The next chapter describes the *Segmental Electrogram* in full.)

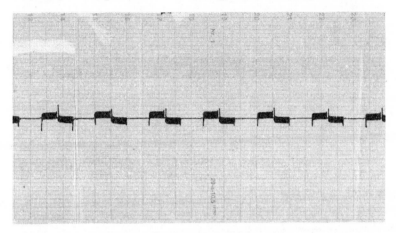

Figure 1: *Segmental Electrogram* recording following electrical stimulation of a female patient with rheumatoid arthritis. She had been on oral steroid drugs for eight years. Notice the flat recording.

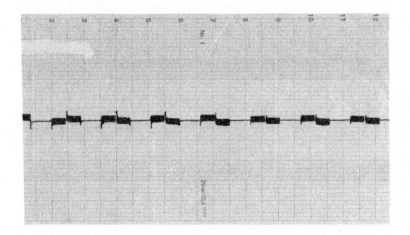

Figure 2: *Segmental Electrogram* recording following electrical stimulation of a male patient with asthma. He had been taking steroids by inhalation for four years. As for Figure 1 note the flat recording.

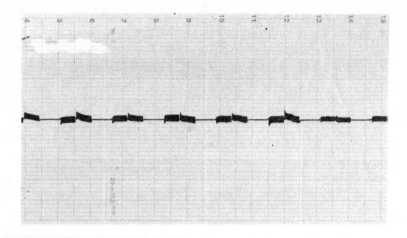

Figure 3: A *Segmental Electrogram* recording before stimulation.

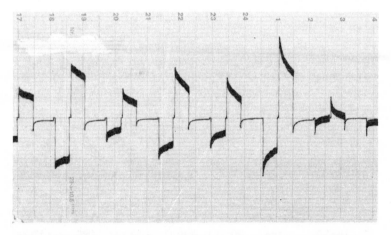

Figure 4: The same *Segmental Electrogram* taken some 5 minutes later, following electrical stimulation. Notice the difference in the height of recordings in all of the sections.

In order for any natural therapy to work, the use of suppressive drugs has to be kept to a minimum, and the patient's state of nutrition including his vitamin and mineral balance has to be looked at carefully.

Causally Directed Therapy

Defining cause is a central issue in bio-electronic regulatory medicine. This is carried out by looking at the body from an electrical point of view. The techniques described in this book are the *segmental electrogram* and the *Vegatest* method. These are capable of much greater sophistication but provide the best available methods at the present time. These systems will be described in detail in the next chapter. They define cause in terms of organ dysfunction, the presence of toxins, psychological factors, environmental influences and the relationship of these factors to each other and their relative importance. Treatment is then based on a causally directed diagnosis. The prime question that BER medicine asks is what caused the illness and how can this best be treated. Conventional medicine tends to ask the question, 'How best can I control my patient's symptoms?' From a practical point of view the latter question must always be addressed to a greater or lesser extent, but it isn't the prime question. In other words pain has to be treated but also the cause must be sought and dealt with.

Stimulatory Therapy

A characteristic of many natural therapies is that they stimulate the body to function more effectively. This is the opposite of conventional approaches. For example, conventional medicine uses various preparations of pancreatic enzymes to treat pancreatic dysfunction. Complementary therapies use herbs, acupuncture point stimulation or a combination of herbal and homoeopathic remedies (known as complex homoeopathy) to stimulate the pancreas to work more efficiently and produce by itself adequate supplies of pancreatic enzymes. Natural therapy stimulates the body to get rid of toxins. This approach is a fundamentally more sensible one than the suppressive approach, as it helps the body utilize all its natural processes in response to any illness. It interests me to note that there are very few drugs in the conventional pharmacopoeia which stimulate any organ to work more efficiently. One exception is Digoxin which is made from a herb anyway, and has been rendered much more toxic by purification and the extraction of its active principle than by giving Digitalis (foxglove) leaf as it occurs naturally. Natural therapeutics, particularly complex homoeopathy, has a real lead over conventional therapeutics in the area of stimulatory therapy.

Preventive Medicine

Modern medicine is constantly criticized for its lack of emphasis on preventive medicine. Unfortunately it does not seem to have the time or energy as it looks as if it might be creating more problems than it is solving. Alternative therapies offer a practical approach to preventive medicine. These involve environmental measures such as the avoidance of chemical pollution, good nutrition with an emphasis on organic food and an adequate supply of vitamins and minerals. A pursuit of psychological health using a wide spectrum of techniques such as autogenic training for stress reduction, and physical fitness by regular exercise such as jogging and swimming are important features of the preventive view as looked at by the natural therapies. Conventional medicine only adequately follows up the exercise dimension of the preventive approach to good health.

All preventive measures demand some active participation from the patient and there is evidence that the opinion leaders, the self-explorers, are actively following a number of the preventative measures mentioned above. The majority of the population, however, cannot be bothered and would much prefer 'a pill for every ill' and to opt out of any personal responsibility for health. Only continued social change along the lines mentioned in Chapter 1 will change this situation.

Conclusion
The predominantly symptomatic approach of conventional medicine deserves to be severely criticized, and perhaps I have spent too much of this chapter labouring this point. However, as this is the status quo, the point needs to be made forcibly. The suppressive measures of conventional medicine are, however, necessary in certain situations and often they can be life-saving. BER medicine provides the beginnings of a viable causally orientated system of medicine, but it is in its early stages of development. It shows every sign of being superior to conventional approaches, both conceptually and practically, but is very short of research input. With a change in public perception of modern medicine this situation may be remedied, and with it we have the possibility of a medicine which is truly objective and causally directed.

5. Bio-electronic Regulatory Techniques, the Segmental Electrogram and the Vegatest Method

New Methods of Diagnosis — the Concept of Energetic Pathology

Most scientists would accept that any biological event is fundamentally an electrical change of one sort or another. We also all accept the reality of invisible radiations passing through the air which can be picked up on a radio or a television set. If the notion that radio waves, or indeed invisible waves of any sort which are packed with informational content, had been suggested to us prior to the invention of radio or television, then most of us would have difficulty in accepting this, very many would dismiss the idea as impossible and very few would at least allow the possibility of their existence.

At the present time we are in a similar position regarding the idea of energetic pathology. Briefly this postulates that the first thing to go wrong in the body is an electrical change. Only when this electrical (energetic) change has been present for a considerable period of time does actual physical organic change in the body begin to occur.

Conventional investigations, such as X-ray examination, the EMI scanner and more recently Nuclear Magnetic Resonance (NMR) all look at structure in the body, albeit in some cases in extraordinary detail (NMR), yet these investigations remain, in the conceptual sense, structural. The energetic (electrical) properties of a tissue or organ are not considered to be important. The view of those practising alternative medicine is that energetic parameters are of primary importance. The implication is that all biological events are basically electrical changes, usually of an ionic nature, and if these are abnormal and continue for long enough then eventually structural change will ensue, which of course will show up when looked at by the conventional methods mentioned. If pathological change can be detected at an energetic stage, then diagnosis can be made much earlier, also pathology at this stage is more easily reversible than when a 'lump' has already appeared. Unfortunately many doctors still consider this view to be nonsense. This is perhaps related to the emphasis in medical training on the disciplines of biology and biochemistry. If doctors were physicists then the alternative view would appear to be more scientific. This is an interesting observation, especially for the legions of doctors who wield the word 'scientific' in defence of their narrow view and against an unorthodox approach.

The observation that structural change in the body ensues following pre-existing long-standing electrical change is repeatedly confirmed by BER techniques. The electrical pathological change initially produces very fine disturbances in the function of the area over which it is acting. As time progresses the functional change produced in this way slowly becomes more marked and eventually causes organic damage.

Conventional tests for organ dysfunction, such as liver function tests (a range of blood tests usually) are hopelessly crude and are unable to detect the subtle functional changes produced by energetic pathology. For example a car engine which isn't tuned properly will only show a slight decrease in performance (function) when under strain, but the engine and all its parts will show no detectable physical change (structure) if examined using the most painstaking of methods available.

From a practical point of view the consideration of energetic pathology is fundamental to BER medicine, and is in many ways its most important contribution to conventional medicine. When pathology is only detected at the stage when organic damage is present then treatment is much less likely to be effective, as in many cases the horse has already bolted. However, if pathology is detected at the energetic stage then the illness is potentially much more reversible, and by implication curable. The findings of BER medicine indicate that electrical (energetic) pathology often pre-dates actual structural damage by many years. Therefore as the ideas and technology used in BER medicine are developed, further researched, and improved we may well have the possibility of early diagnosis at the energetic level in a way that very few have dreamt of at the present time. This is truly an exciting, but I maintain, a realistic goal.

Structural change in the body clearly also produces electrical change, but often this only shows up when the body is stressed, usually with a low voltage pulse. Without stressing the body electrically, it appears to compensate very effectively for any organic change which may be present. It is highly probable that illness starts in an electrical sense, both inside and outside the body, in the body's energy field. This may extend several inches from the body's surface. The final chapter explores ways of exploiting this apparently futuristic and fanciful idea.

The rest of this chapter will describe what, in my view, are the most successful and efficient methods available at the present time for making an energetic diagnosis from a causal point of view, the aim being to define causes and then treat them. In practice this turns out to be a more successful and long-lasting way of treating chronic illness than concentrating therapeutically on symptom suppression. The methods described here are the *Segmental Electrogram* and the *Vegatest* method. These techniques are still in their early stages of development, but are the best tools available in BER medicine at the present time. In many cases when using these methods it is possible to reach a causal diagnosis, but this may take a number of appointments in order to see any chronic illness in all its causal complexity. In other words illness can be compared to an onion when looked at using BER diagnostic techniques, and as the illness improves another layer of the onion skin is removed revealing the next, and so on until the causal chain becomes clear. In a number of cases the cause is obvious from the first examination, but in some cases no obvious cause can be detected. Developments in BER techniques should reduce the size of the latter group. In other words these methods make the best possible attempt at causal diagnosis at the present time.

The Segmental Electrogram[1]
This is the most objective BER technique, and of all these methods the easiest to relate to conventional diagnosis. Therefore it provides the main point of contact between BER and conventional medicine.

Description of equipment
The *SEG* records skin impedance (which equals a combination of the resistive effect of the skin and the capacitative resistance of internal body structures) over eight body quadrants (head left and right, chest left and right, abdomen left and right, pelvis left and right[1]). The recording electrodes are placed on specific body areas. The numbers refer to the eight body quadrants. For example, quadrant 1 records the impedance with time across the left forehead

and left C7 electrodes at the level of the seventh cervical vertebra. A 13 cycle per second (Hertz) exploratory voltage (too small to be felt by the patient as it is only 2 volts) is applied via circular silver electrodes over each quadrant in sequence. The response in terms of change of impedance with time over each quadrant is recorded on a moving paper recorder (Figures 6 and 7).

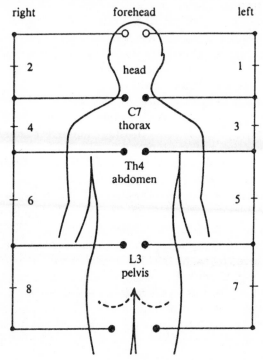

Figure 5:   Diagram of electrode placement for the *Segmental Electrogram.*

As the diameter of the electrodes is relatively large (6 cm), it can be assumed that the skin resistance beneath the area of the electrodes is more or less equal over the whole electrode area. This means that the change of the exploratory voltage which is subsequently recorded as a *Segmental Electrogram* recording, is largely brought about by the impedance of the major internal organs situated in each quadrant. It therefore serves as a useful pointer to organ dysfunction. For example, as the liver is the largest organ situated in the abdomen right quadrant, this part of the *SEG* tells us something about liver function, similarly the lungs in the

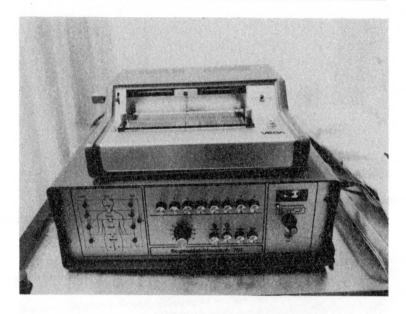

Figure 6:   The *Segmental Electrogram* equipment.

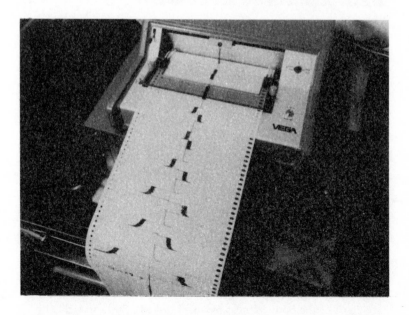

Figure 7:   The *Segmental Electrogram Recorder* making a typical recording.

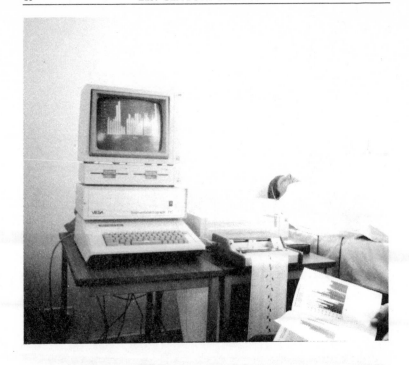

Figure 8: The computerized Segmental Electrogram.

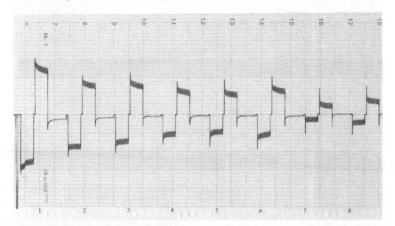

Figure 9: A typical *Segmental Electrogram* recording. Each quadrant is labelled from 1 through to 8 and below this the relevant part of the body is indicated. 1=head left, 2=head right, 3= chest left, 4=chest right, 5=abdomen left, 6=abdomen right, 7=pelvis left, 8=pelvis right.

chest segments, and so on. Recently the *Segmental Electrogram* has been computerized on an *Apple* computer (see Figure 8).

A typical Segmental Electrogram recording is shown in Figure 9. Each quadrant is labelled on this recording and each refers to the quadrants detailed in Figure 5. Generally speaking, the height of the deflection above the central zero line should be slightly longer than that below the zero line. The first part of each quadrant recording records the change produced by passing a 13 cycles per second 2-volt exploratory current into each quadrant in a negative polarity. This is then repeated in the positive polarity which is shown in each quadrant recording by the segment above the zero line. The next section of the recording is the so called reverse current which records electrical changes taking place after the exploratory voltage has been passed. All these factors are shown in detail in Figure 10. Generally speaking the recording in each quadrant should be of a similar amptitude to all the other quadrants. This is, in fact, rarely seen but is what a normal recording should look like. Also the reverse current should remain below the zero line and the sloping part of each recording both above and below the zero line should form a nice triangular shape. The computerized *Segmental Electrogram* compares the mathematical proportions between each deflection of the recording in each quadrant and converts these into histograms (bar graphs) which are shown in Figure 11.

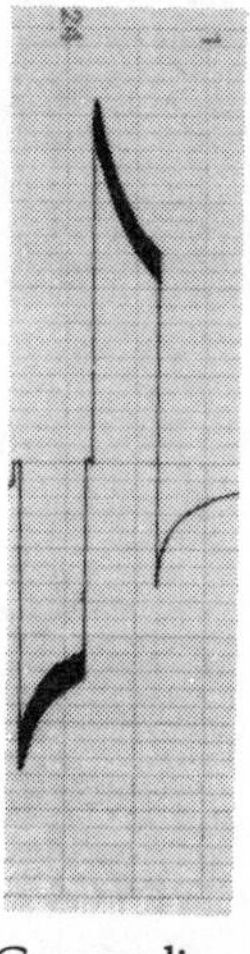

Figure 10: Detail of an *SEG* recording from a single quadrant. The first segment below the zero line is called a negative impulse packet, that which follows above the zero line is the positive impulse packet, followed by the reverse current.

COMPUTER-SEG according to DR.DR. H.W. Schimmel　　at February 1985

DR. JULIAN KENYON

recorded at 31 5 85　　1 00 P .M.

surname

first name

street

town

date of birth

chronicity factor		disturbance field factor	
head left	60	head left	0
head right	20	head right	65
thorax left	60	thorax left	0
thorax right	55	thorax right	15
abdomen left	55	abdomen left	0
abdomen right	50	abdomen right	15
pelvis left	50	pelvis left	65
pelvis right	40	pelvis right	65

According to the SEG-reading, taking the RPN-factor into consideration
an average is calculated:
a tendecy to l i m i t e d regulation.

The relevant energy situation refers in its bioelectronic components to:
t o o l o w a level.

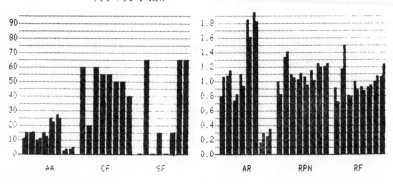

REC	AA		AR		RPN		RF	
	before	after	before	after	before	after	before	after
1	11	15	.79	1.06	.99	.82	.91	.72
2	15	16	1.07	1.14	1.33	1.41	1.17	1.5
3	10	11	.73	.82	1.08	1.05	.81	.8
4	15	13	1.09	.93	1.02	1.11	1	.88
5	25	22	1.84	1.61	1.06	.95	.92	.87
6	28	25	2.03	1.82	1.14	1.01	.92	.95
7	2	4	.16	.28	1.25	1.19	1	1.07
8	4	5	.25	.34	1.21	1.25	1.06	1.23

Figure 11:　A typical computerized *Segmental Electrogram* recording.

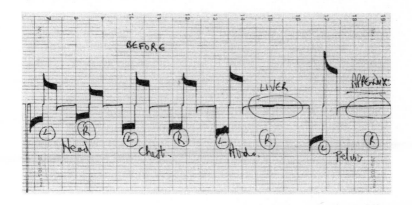

Figure 12: An *SEG* from a nine-year-old boy with chronic appendicitis. The symptoms were poor school performance, general malaise, and wheat and milk intolerance. The appendix is shown in the far right-hand quadrant recording over the pelvis on the right.

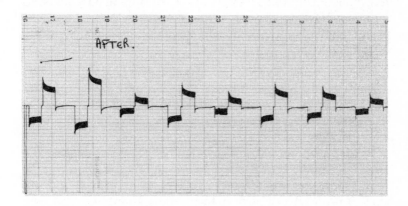

Figure 13: Follow-up *SEG* on the same patient shown in Figure 12, some months afterwards, following complex homoeopathic therapy. Notice the improvement in the 6th and 8th quadrants.

Examples of Diseases Revealed by the Segmental Electrogram but Not Shown by Conventional Investigative Techniques

1. *Chronic Appendicitis.* The majority of current surgical opinion does not recognize the existence of chronic appendicitis. X-ray and conventional scanning techniques show no consistent abnormality which could fit such a diagnosis. The *SEG* shows that chronic appendicitis does exist. Figure 12 is from a young boy with chronic appendicitis (which shows up on the *SEG*). The parameters all improved, indicating that it would be likely to respond to conservative measures (complex homoeopathy), which in fact it did as shown by the follow-up *SEG* recording in Figure 13.

This patient's symptoms were poor school performance, general malaise, and wheat and milk intolerance. There was nothing in the history or examination of the patient to suggest a diagnosis of chronic appendicitis. All his symptoms cleared up following treatment.

Figure 14 is an *SEG* from a 50-year-old male patient complaining of severe malaise, itching eyes and vague abdominal discomfort for twelve years. The recording shows chronic appendicitis, and the post stimulation recording (Figure 15) shows a worsening of all parameters. In simple terms the deflections are less on the post stimulation recording (Figure 15) than on the pre-stimulation recording (Figure 14). This patient needed surgical removal of his appendix. He responded only partially to conservative management using complex homoeopathy but recovered fully after the removal of the appendix.

2. *Causal Chains.* The *SEG* reveals fascinating causal relationships in illnesses which can be difficult to understand. To illustrate this point Figure 16 is a recording from a patient with urticaria (an intermittent red raised blotchy rash which itches and is considered to be of allergic origin).

In her past history this patient had had recurrent sinusitis and tonsillitis (shown in quadrant 1 recording over the left side of the head as irregular impulse packets). This led to many episodes of chronic bronchitis (shown on the third quadrant recording over the left side of the chest by an abnormality on the positive impulse packet), for which she had taken regular courses of broad spectrum antibiotics. These in turn had altered the normal colonic bacteria leading to altered bowel function and increased permeability of the intestinal mucous membrane (the lining membrane of the bowel). This is shown by an irregular positive impulse packet in the seventh quadrant recording over the left side of the pelvis. This

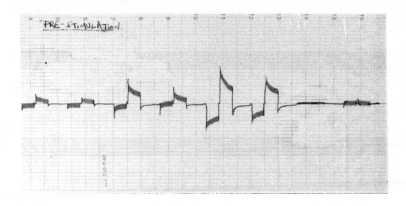

Figure 14: Segmental Electrogram from a 50-year-old male patient complaining of severe malaise, itching eyes and vague abdominal discomfort for 12 years. Notice the low amptitude recordings in the pelvic quadrants (7 and 8).

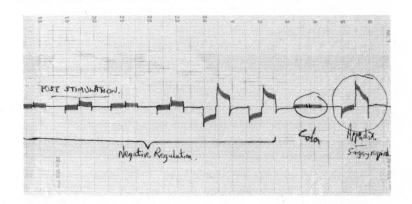

Figure 15: Post stimulation *SEG* from the same patient as in Figure 14. Notice the reduced deflections on most of the quadrants compared to the pre-stimulation recording and also the appearance of irregular impulse packets in the far right hand side quadrant recording over the right side of the pelvis.

had led to the re-absorption of toxins from the intestines which then passed into the liver circulation, eventually ending up at the liver causing dysfunction in this organ (this is shown by irregular positive and negative impulse packets in the sixth quadrant recording over the right side of the abdomen). Her urticaria was brought on by

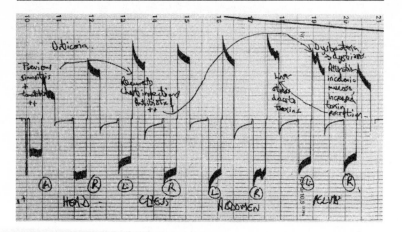

Figure 16:   A recording from a 26-year-old female patient
with urticaria.

contact with various substances to which she was allergic,
particularly milk and dairy products, but the chain of events as
revealed by the *SEG* showed the underlying cause of these allergies
which in turn produced her urticaria.

Treatment was directed at normalizing the bacteria in the colon
which had been destroyed by the antibiotics given many years
earlier for her recurrent sinusitis and tonsillitis. This was done by
giving preparations containing normal live colonic bacteria. Liver
function was improved by avoiding fats and alcohol and stimulating
the liver with appropriate complex homoeopathic preparations (see

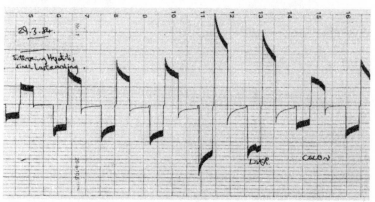

Figure 17:   The follow-up *SEG* recording made on the same patient
as shown in Figure 16.

Chapter 8). Lastly, the patient had to be de-toxified from the antibiotics (which had remained to a certain extent in the liver). This was achieved by giving a nosode (a homoeopathic dilution) of a mixture of antibiotics. It is of interest that conventional liver function tests were normal in this patient. On this treatment programme she made a full recovery as shown by a subsequent recording (Figure 17) in spite of an intervening infectious hepatitis (shown by an irregular negative impulse packet in the sixth quadrant recording over the right side of the abdomen).

Many different causal chains have been found underlying most chronic illnesses investigated with the *SEG*, with a consequent novel view of their causation and appropriate treatment. These findings imply that conventional views of much chronic illness are simplistic and therapy is often inappropriate, even though it may well work, for example the use of antihistamines or steroids in urticaria.

What does the normal SEG look like?
Strictly speaking there is no such thing as a normal *SEG*, as everybody is dealing with many past and present pathological insults of various sorts. Therefore total health in an energetic sense is theoretically impossible. From the point of view of the doctor-patient relationship this is a fortunate thing as it means that the final decision in terms of patient management is a clinical one and does not rest with the machine. With an energetic (electrical) approach to diagnosis as exemplified by the *SEG* the machine will never take over the all-important human element of medicine. It therefore has its own inbuilt safeguard, in contrast to some conventional methods of investigation in which the procedure itself can assume primary importance.

Conclusion
The *SEG* provides a fascinating insight into chronic disease and calls into question the idea of putting diseases into neat diagnostic boxes. This will be discussed more fully later in this chapter. However, the SEG only tells us in which quadrant the abnormality is found, it doesn't indicate which organ is involved. From many years of experience in BER medicine the following organs are the most likely to be involved if the relevant *SEG* quadrant recording is abnormal.

Head quadrants (1 and 2)	Most commonly the sinuses, followed by tonsils in young adults or the teeth in older people.

Chest quadrants (3 and 4)	The diaphragm is most likely to show up here as the stressed organ, followed by the lung and clearly the heart if the left chest quadrant is abnormal.
Abdominal quadrants (5 and 6)	On the left side the pancreas shows up as being the most commonly stressed organ and on the right side the liver. In some cases, however, the kidney, small intestine, stomach, duodenum or gall bladder may show up as the most stressed organ, although this is less common than stress of the pancreas or liver.
Pelvic quadrants (7 and 8)	The most commonly stressed organ to show up in the pelvis is the colon, particularly on the left side. On the right side the appendix shows up most commonly. Other organs may also be involved such as the bladder, uterus, ovaries and prostate gland, although these are less often affected than the colon.

Therefore the *SEG* provides limited information in terms of which organs are involved. It does, however, enable many chronic illnesses to be worked out in a causal chain sense.

The next piece of equipment provides the extra detail not shown by the *SEG* in order to reach a complete causal diagnosis. This is the *Vegatest* machine.

The Vegatest Method

Introduction
The *Vegatest* method relies on changes in the resistance to the flow of electricity over acupuncture points on the ends of fingers or toes, brought about by bringing particular substances, in glass phials, into series in the circuit. In practice a tiny direct current voltage of 0.87 of a volt is applied via a ball-shaped silver electrode on to a point on the end of a finger or toe. The patient holds a silver-plated cylinder to complete the circuit. The electricity flows from

the electrode, seen in Figure 18, which is applied to a point over

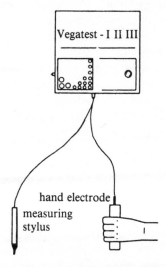

Figure 18:   Diagrammatic representation of the *Vegatest* method.

the end of the finger or toe, and then passes via various complicated pathways through the body and out by the hand-held electrode. The device is shown in operation in Figure 19.

History of the Vegatest Method

The *Vegatest* method evolved from techniques for measuring acupuncture points developed by a German doctor, Dr Reinholdt Voll in the early 1950s. Most of the credit for pioneering these techniques is due to Dr Voll. He decided to test out whether electrical measurement of acupuncture points on specific meridians bore any relation to the organs to which the measured point belonged, in other words he decided to use the names of the meridians in a much more literal sense than has ever been accepted in classical Chinese acupuncture. He postulated, for example, that at least some points on the large intestine meridian may represent specific parts of the large intestine itself, and may reflect the function of these areas depending on the measurements made over these points. There does seem to be some truth in this idea and it was tested by measuring many patients with known pathology in particular organs, and seeing which points showed abnormal readings.

The cardinal abnormality shown on a measured point is the indicator drop. The acupuncture point is electrically negative with respect to surrounding skin. The positive side of the measurement circuit is placed on the point via a point probe (see Figures 18, 19a and 19b). As opposite charges cancel each other out, then in order for the reading on the point to remain steady the electro-motive force (measured in volts) of the acupuncture point must exactly balance that of the measurement voltage. In order to do this the electro-motive force of the point (which behaves rather like a battery) must be constantly replenished, and this is what is probably happening in practice, as if this were not the case the indicator on the voltmeter would start to fall; this is the so-called indicator drop. It is assumed that this replenishing of charge to the battery-like acupuncture point is produced by a flow of bio-electric energy moving along the appropriate meridian connected to the acupuncture point under examination, and this is what replenishes the energy at the point. This is illustrated diagrammatically in Figure 20.

Dr Voll built up a highly complicated diagnostic system based

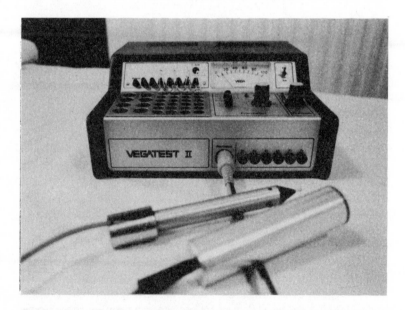

Figure 19a: The *Vegatest* device in operation. The 'honeycomb' seen on the top surface of the *Vegatest* device just to the left of the indicator dial, and on the diagram in *Figure 18* is connected in series into the circuit; in other words electricity flows in from one side of the honeycomb, then through the honeycomb and out the other side. Substances to be tested are placed in one of the holes in the honeycomb.

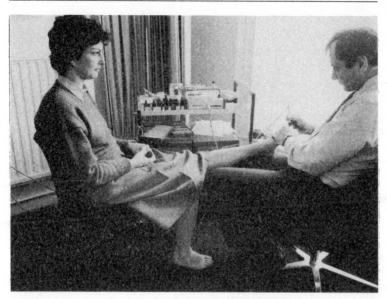

Figure 19b: The *Vegatest* device in operation. The hand-held electrode is applied to a point on the tip of the toe, the patient holds the hand-held electrode as shown.

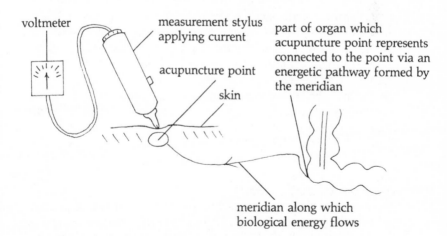

Figure 20:   Diagram of bio-energetic changes at acupuncture points being caused by a flow of energy along an acupuncture meridian.

upon the acupuncture meridian system.[2] He then discovered that if he put medications into series in the circuit (into the honeycomb) which could help the patient's problem then all the previously recorded indicator drops would disappear and all points would record 50 on the indicator scale if the appropriate remedy were in the honeycomb at the time of measurement. This was the birth of medicine testing which is a corner-stone of bio-electronic regulatory medicine. This breakthrough heralded a new era for homoeopathy. For the first time the effects of these remedies, and indeed those of allopathic drugs, allergens, foods or chemicals to which a patient might be sensitive, could be measured. This took a lot of guesswork out of homoeopathy and improved the effectiveness of this system of medicine in patients with chronic disease. This approach spread rapidly in Germany, but oddly enough little interest was shown by classical homoepaths outside Germany. Voll's technique showed that more than one remedy was nearly always needed in order to normalize the readings made on a patient, which is contrary to the dogma of classical homoeopathy (see Chapter 8).

The enormous advantages that Voll's system gave both to diagnosis and treatment were countered to an extent by the enormous complexity of the method. Often many points have to be measured and then it would not be clear how to organize the diagnostic information obtained into rank order of importance. As a consequence examinations are often long drawn out and very tiring for the practitioner. Dr Helmut Schimmel was one of many doctors looking for an easier and less complex way round. He thought that instead of taking the acunpuncture point itself as being the main diagnostic indicator, as in the Voll system (i.e. a large intestine point refers to a large intestine problem), why not use one point and take as the diagnostic indicator ampoules containing homoeopathic extracts of normal mammalian organs, such as an ampoule consisting of homoeopathic extract of the large intestine acting as the main indicator for problems in the large intestine.[1] This was the birth, in the early 1970s, of the *Vegatest* system.

Using the Vegatest method[3]

The equipment used in this technique is very similar to that used in Dr Voll's method. Electrically it is a Wheatstone bridge circuit (a standard electrical circuit for comparing resistances). In the *Vegatest* method the main indicator of an abnormality is the so-called disorder control. This describes the phenomenon of a lower reading being obtained when a substance is put into series in the circuit (in the honeycomb) which indicates an abnormality in the patient, for example in the liver if the substance is a homoeopathic extract of liver. A lower reading would be expected anyway if the substance which is put into circuit is a poison — something which is allergenic to the patient or a poisonous chemical. Therefore liver dysfunction can be ascertained simply by placing a homoeopathic ampoule of liver in the circuit and then re-measuring the same point. If the reading is lower then this indicates liver dysfunction.

In Dr Voll's system the same conclusion would be reached by measuring over a liver point and seeing if an indicator drop is present or not. If it is then the diagnosis is the same, i.e. there is liver dysfunction present. The *Vegatest* method is technically more difficult to carry out than the Voll method, but this disadvantage is more than made up for by its rapidity and simplicity. Of all the BER techniques the *Vegatest* method is, for the reasons mentioned, the method of choice. However both the Voll and *Vegatest* methods are weak links in the system of BER techniques. They both rely on operator skill, and this is more critical with the *Vegatest* method than with the Voll technique. They are both prone to operator error, the Voll technique less than the *Vegatest* method. In many ways they are similar to using a stethoscope, in that (as my Professor of Medicine told me when I misinterpreted a heart murmur) the most important part is the bit between the ears! In the *Vegatest* and the Voll methods the operator is of major importance. To an extent both techniques have a subjective element (this can be considered as an observer effect). This is a problem which must be faced fairly and squarely and is discussed in detail in Chapter 6. There is a possibility that more sophisticated systems will be developed in the future which will be able to reach a more objective diagnosis in terms of subtle electrical change in the body. The final chapter looks forward to these methods.

The pre-tests and organ tests
The diagnostic system in the *Vegatest* method is divided into two parts. The first consists of pre-tests which attempt to define the pathological terrain. For example, they ask questions by means of specific homoeopathic test ampoules placed in circuit as to whether there is a toxin (poison) present, if geopathic stress is relevant or if there is a focus, as well as other relevant questions. The identity of the specific ampoules for asking each question has been reached by trial and error. Many are homoeopathic potencies of important trace elements in the body, such as zinc or chromium.

Organ dysfunction is tested by means of homoeopathic potencies of normal mammalian organs. Lastly a group of pre-tests is used in order to structure the diagnostic information into a meaningful whole. For example these ask questions such as 'which is the most stressed organ?' and 'is the problem predominantly toxic or mainly a psychological problem?' and so on. The aim is to reach a causally directed organ-based diagnosis as well as to identify additional important factors such as the presence of a focus and other factors which will be mentioned later in this chapter. The secret of the system is diagnosis. It is much easier to design treatment around an accurate diagnosis reached in this manner.

Electrical stressing of the body
Just as in the *SEG* method the body needs to be stressed electrically before measurement. This is done using a piezo-electric spark generator (producing a spark of about 4000 volts) applied over the terminal points of particular meridians (see Figure 21). This ensures that as much of the clinical picture as possible becomes recordable following electrical stressing.

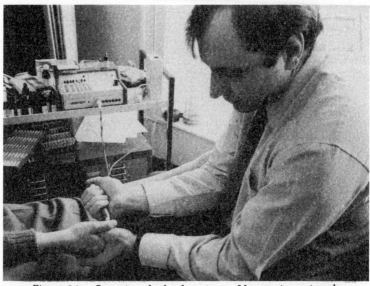

Figure 21:   Stressing the body prior to *Vegatesting* using the PM 2000 over the acupuncture points lymph 1 and allergy 1 bilaterally. (These are spread points described by Dr Voll.)

Organ Stress — a New Concept
The idea of organ stress or of medications claiming to improve

organ function is not a new one. It carries the unfortunate stigma of the claims made on patent medicine bottles and sounds unscientific. In order to validate the idea of organ stress (which is synonymous in this context with organ dysfunction) we must first look at conventional methods of looking at organ function. The liver is a good example. Assessments of liver function involve many tests, ranging from blood investigations, and biopsy (an examination of small pieces of tissue taken from the liver), to modern sophisticated scanning techniques (such as nuclear magnetic resonance). These look at one particular aspect of liver function, such as the blood level of a particular enzyme, or the reduced ability of the liver to metabolize (use up and destroy) specific substances in the body. In reality, however, liver function is manifest by the simultaneous activity of a vast range of specific functions, a sort of Gestalt of the liver. This therefore questions the usefulness of individual estimations of specific aspects of liver function but nevertheless they do remain useful and valid. All conventional current methods of estimating organ function are firmly in the reductionist conceptual mould (see Chapter 3).

Looking at the electrical activity of the liver as a whole is probably a much more useful method of looking at organ dysfunction and certainly complements the conventional tests previously mentioned. In other words a parameter is taken which represents the Gestalt of the myriad of specific liver functions all going on at the particular moment when the measurement is made. In practice this turns out to be a highly sensitive measure of what has been called, in BER medicine, organ stress or dysfunction. Organ stress implies a number of possibilities such as that one or a number of specific liver functions are deranged (uncommon except in significant physical organ damage), or that a number of individual functions are slightly below par and as a consequence their relationships with each other are slightly out of balance, (this is probably the most common situation when BER techniques detect organ stress). Therefore there will not always be a correspondence between conventional tests of organ dysfunction and liver organ stress as defined by BER techniques. This makes the BER idea of organ stress difficult to evaluate by conventional methods and necessitates the development of a whole range of new technology in order to validate it scientifically (see Chapter 15). The concept only remains unscientific in so far as this new technology has not yet been developed. However, from a conceptual point of view it is an idea which falls firmly into the holistic camp, and from a theoretical point of view concurs with much of modern physics (see Chapter 3).

Focal Illness, an Old Idea Re-assessed

The concept of focal infection (that is infection localized to a small area of the body, such as a tooth root) was fashionable in conventional medicine up until World War II. A focus is defined as the presence in the connective tissue of non-absorbable material. This may be a bacteria or virus (most commonly parts of the dead viral or bacterial body which are usually proteins and are highly reactive in the body), a foreign material such as dental amalgam or metal from an old gunshot wound, or a toxin (such as pesticides, insecticides, industrial chemicals, etc). Before the Second World War it was not uncommon to recommend that patients with rheumatoid arthritis should have all their teeth removed because of the possibility that focal dental infection was an important cause of their illness. A number of rheumatoids recovered following dental clearance, but most noticed no difference and lost all their teeth to boot! The idea of focal infection therefore fell from grace and was deemed largely invalid. This is a good example of an idea with validity which was shown by the science of the day to be ineffective. However, BER techniques enable those patients whose rheumatoid arthritis could be helped by dental treatment to locate which particular teeth need removal or specialized dental work. This is a new way of looking at an old idea, with every possibility of it now being proven valid as a result. It is interesting to note how misdirected scientific proof can be, simply because the nature of a phenomenon is not adequately understood. BER medicine certainly encourages a more open-minded attitude to the 'science' of the past and present.

Foci are usually very small anatomically, and produce their effects over a very long period of time. They seem to act like the proverbial spanner in the works, producing a very small energetic disturbance, but which acts over many years, thus ultimately producing an effect disproportionate to its size. Most foci are found in the teeth, tonsils, sinuses, appendix, gall bladder and prostate. However any organ may act as a focus. BER diagnoses always take into account the presence of foci, and their relative importance.

Geopathic Stress

BER medicine takes account of the possibility that people can be affected adversely by the geomagnetic aspects of the environment in which they live. The existence of this situation is called geopathic stress. The implication is that very small changes in the earth's geomagnetic field acting over a number of years can produce effects detrimental to health. The scientific verification of this concept is practically non-existent, but the biological effects of very small magnetic fields have been very well known and extensively researched for some time.[4] The concept of geopathic stress is beloved of many lay healers where it is given the name 'ley line stress'. It is an idea which can be traced back to antiquity.

I have absolutely no doubt that geopathic stress is a genuine and clinically important concept. Many patients will not respond to treatment, particularly any that relies on the manipulation of biological energy such as most of the natural therapies, unless any pre-existing geopathic stress is removed. The methods for doing this, at our present minimal understanding of this important concept, depend on making use of the services of a dowser (water diviner). The methods used by different dowsers for the correction of geopathic stress vary widely; some are notably more successful than others. Removal of a pre-existing geopathic stress and the subsequent improvement of the patient is clinically impressive, and has left me and many of my colleagues in no doubt as to its validity.

My own definition of geopathic stress is that it is a minute change in the ambient geomagnetic field, usually brought about by factors that alter the electrical conductivity of the earth in the area under consideration. The factors that most often cause this are geological faults in the earth's crust, underground water, particularly wells, mining and building works. Power cables (overhead or underground) may also produce similar effects. It is likely that future technology will enable us to study geopathic stress in a more objective and scientific manner.

Toxicity

BER techniques show that a major cause of chronic illness is toxicity (poisoning) from a variety of sources, such as insecticides or pesticides. The findings are that rather than excrete toxins, the body appears to store them, particularly in fat cells and in the liver, where they may remain locked away for many years causing slow, insidious but relentless damage to the body. Modern research into chemical poisoning confirms the view that toxins tend to accumulate in the tissues.

Causal Chains

BER medicine shows that disease does not exist in isolation in the body: inevitably illness will spread and involve more and more organs the longer it is present. The *SEG* and the *Vegatest* methods allow the progression of disease to be defined and a causal chain to be worked out. This is of some practical importance as therapy directed at the beginning of the causal chain is more likely to be successful than when it is directed at any other part of the sequence. Experienced practitioners will only need to use the *Segmental Electrogram* in complicated cases, as it has been found that there are a limited number of causal chains, and in experienced hands the *Vegatest* method is usually all that is necessary to determine which causal chain is operating. The *SEG* remains useful as an objective recording of the patient's energetic state at the time of examination.

Treatment

Once the diagnosis has been made the direction which treatment should take is clear. For example, a focus may need surgical treatment, such as appendicectomy or tooth extraction. It may, however, respond to conservative treatment if the patient has a good regulatory capacity, and therefore has the ability to react positively to therapy. If toxins are present than appropriate nosodes (homoeopathic dilutions of toxins) can be given (see Chapter 8). The stressed organs can be treated with combinations of herbal and homoeopathic remedies (known as complex homoeopathy) which are organ targeted (see Chapter 8). Naturopathic measures may also be advised. These may include the avoidance of fats and alcohol if the liver is the most stressed organ, or of refined carbohydrates if the pancreas is the most stressed. Complex homoeopathy is the mainstay of treatment when using BER medicine with other measures added as necessary. The remedies can be balanced electrically against the appropriate acupuncture points or organ ampoules of the stressed organs using the *Vegatest* method. The combination of remedies which when in the honeycomb electrically balances all the abnormalities found during diagnosis are likely to be those which will be effective as treatment. The *Vegatest* method determines whether or not the treatment will be effective and tolerated by the patient. The various responses to treatment will be discussed in detail in Chapter 11.

Conclusion

The *SEG* and the *Vegatest* give a fascinating insight into the causation of many chronic illnesses. They also allow appropriate and effective treatment to be determined. They are the beginnings of what may well turn out to be the foundations of the medicine of the future.

BER medicine shows that current concepts of disease are outdated. Conventional medicine attempts to put illnesses into neat diagnostic boxes, such as rheumatoid arthritis, or ulcerative colitis, etc. BER techniques show that in reality many chronic diseases are a collection of widely differing causes, therefore to classify as we do is misleading. Often our classification of chronic illness is based on particular symptom complexes, which again illustrates the current preoccupation with symptoms rather than causes. It is far more useful to define disease in terms of causation rather than by its characteristic symptom complex, as this helps in deciding where therapy should be directed. Also the same set of causes can produce widely different illnesses in different people.

If illnesses, particularly chronic diseases, were defined in causal terms such as by a causal chain, and the relative importance of psychological, toxic and other causes was defined, then the attitude of both doctor and patient might be subtly different. I have always been interested by how many doctors, myself included, strive by all means available to put a patient into a diagnostic slot. The implication from both points of view is that labelling the illness is somehow therapeutic, and that once the disease has been classified nothing else need be done.

The habit of classifying illnesses into separate categories has been carried over into the way medicine is constituted. Specialism is the name of the game. At the time of writing there are nearly fifty separate specialities recognized by the British National Health Service; when it began in 1948 there were less than fifteen. In the eyes of the various private health insurance schemes only specialist treatment is considered worthy of recognition, and a more general approach is, by implication, second class. This has led to a scramble for specialism with the inevitable consequences of a narrow view and vested interest. This can and does in some cases lead to tragically inappropriate treatment. BER techniques clearly show that disease does not occur in isolation, so the idea of a liver specialist, for example, becomes untenable. It is likely that the doctor of the future will be generalist in approach but specialist in capability.

6. The Psyche in Medicine

Discussion of the psyche (the mind) in terms of psychiatric illness is perfectly acceptable within the domain of psychiatry, even though the conventional therapeutic approach often centres around tinkering with brain neurochemistry. It is when an extension of the influence of the psyche beyond these realms is suggested that causes much difficulty and indeed some hostility. The *Vegatest* method touches on this area as it has a subjective element to it. Scientific materialism has all but slammed the door on subjective phenomena, yet they remain an important part of our everyday experience. As a consequence some attempt to explain the scientific nature of the subjective side of the *Vegatest* method is called for. This topic brings into question many of our methods of studying the body and its response to treatment. But first a word about psychological therapies.

Psychological Therapies

The *Vegatest* method is able to pick out patients in whom psychological causes are of primary importance. The astute physician is able to do the same thing by simply relying on a sixth sense, having no need of recourse to any machine. The argument rests on how the psychological problem is dealt with. All too often conventional psychiatry relies on mood-changing drugs which remove many of the obvious psychological symptoms shown by the patient. This rarely achieves anything in the long run and is tantamount to pushing an iceberg under water. Unfortunately drug-based approaches are increasingly being used to treat everyday human misery, which has been elevated to the status of a disease.

In my experience psychological problems need a psychological approach, using techniques such as counselling or psychotherapy which attempt to identify and treat the psychological root problem.

All too often this is long drawn out work with worthwhile rewards for those who can stay the course. Nevertheless it represents a fundamentally better approach than suppressive drug therapy. Relaxation techniques can be useful in some cases to help patients cope with stress, and of the many methods available autogenic training[1] and hypnosis[2] seem to be the most effective. Unfortunately stress reduction is a relatively superficial approach, and many patients need a more painstaking, analytical approach.

The relatively recent rise of family therapy[3] parallels the increasing interest in holistic approaches to other areas of medicine. Family therapy, simply stated, looks at the way those closest to the patient relate both to him and his illness, and in so doing see the illness in its true context. In many ways family therapy is a reaction to the failures of psychotherapy, and is showing much promise in patients who for many reasons find it impossible to change in response to a conventional psychotherapeutic approach.

More recently there has been a move to recognize the spiritual aspects of psychological illness,[4] in a non-religious context, thereby implying an increasing acceptance of man's spiritual nature. Generally speaking the vast majority of doctors (and patients) run a mile when the basis of their problem is recognized as being a spiritual one, but there are signs that this may be changing. I view all of the techniques mentioned here, including the recognition of the social aspects of mental illness as being an essential part of the management of psychological problems, and they form an integral part of the new system of medicine which this book forsees. In my experience the majority of my failures in therapy have been due to psychological problems which the patient either will not face up to or which resist all attempts at treatment.

Subjective Aspects of BER Techniques

All BER techniques, except the *SEG*, are partially dependent on the psyche of the practitioner, and to that extent are examples of psychophysical systems. Stated at its baldest this means that to an extent the changes in readings noted are partially psychokinetic (PK) effects (literally 'mind-caused' effects), which may in some cases be observed extra sensorily. To the majority of scientists the existence of any subjective element in measurement makes the phenomenon unscientific. The following discussion attempts to counter this view.

Much of this section deals in detail with the findings of modern physics and their relevance to the psyche, thereby making the possibility that mind can affect living matter more scientifically acceptable. A number of scientists have considered that if quantum physics is the best description of reality available at the present time then it should take account of the psyche. Professor D. F. Lawden[5] of Aston University is notable amongst these. He points out that if the mind is truly a peripheral phenomenon then it will remain as a footnote to any future scientific account of the universe, it will also continue to defy scientific explanation simply because it will lie outside the bounds of science. Yet the most successful mathematical theory of physics, namely quantum theory, demands that the conscious observation of the physical system will instantaneously alter its state and that this disturbance will be propagated to distant parts of the system instantaneously, that is at a speed greater than light.

By way of explanation quantum theory considers that the state of the physical system before an observation is represented by a mechanical device called a state vector, which is very similar to the wave function of quantum physics. This contains within it all possible states which the system might assume when an observation is eventually made. For example consider an experiment to observe the position of a photon (packet of energy) using a fixed photographic plate. Before the observation the photon may be represented by a wave extending over the whole surface of the plate (the so-called wave function). This wave function describes the state vector of the system and this represents the potentiality of the photon for interacting with the plate to produce marks at a definite position. It represents all the possible interactions of the photon and their respective probabilities. The wave extending over the whole surface of the plate indicates that it is possible for the photon to interact anywhere on that surface. As a result of conscious observation the photon actualizes one of these possibilities, thereby excluding all other possibilities of interaction. This is called the collapse of the state vector, i.e. a physical change in the state of the system brought about by observation.

The supposition that this change will be propagated at a speed greater than light, or indeed instantaneously to distant parts of the system, arose from the Einstein, Rosen, Podolsky (ERP) effect.[6] These three physicists put forward a proposition supported by a flawless mathematical proof that if quantum theory were correct then the change in one particle in a two particle system, if observed, would affect its twin simultaneously, even if the two had been widely separated in the meantime. This supposedly implies acausal action outside the space/time dimensions as the effect is instantaneous and independent of distance. The problem from a scientific point of view is that travelling faster than light is impossible as it contradicts the theory of relativity. However a recent experiment carried out by Professor Alain Aspect[7] at the Institute D'optique at Orsay near Paris has confirmed the ERP effect. Aspect and his colleagues at Orsay measured the correlation in the polarization of pairs of photons emitted in certain electron transitions from atoms of calcium and mercury. The plane of polarization of the photon is variable and can only be polarized in the plane either parallel or perpendicular to a defined direction in space. In the experiment two separate photo-detectors were placed on either side of a mercury or calcium source, with a polarizer in between each detector and the mercury or calcium. The polarizers only allowed those photons through which were polarized in one

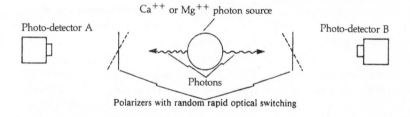

Figure 22: Diagram to explain Aspect's experiment. Aspect's team introduced switches so that the direction of polarization was chosen only at the last possible instant after the photons had left the source. This rules out the objection that the polarizer between photo detector A and the photon source could in some way know the plane of polarization of the polarizer between photo detector B and the photon source.

direction. Aspect then attached a rapid optical switch, switching in a random manner to each polarizer, the switching occurring so rapidly (taking ten nanoseconds, that is, ten thousand millionths of a second) that no signal at the speed of light had time to travel from one detector to the other. What they found was that photons detected simultaneously did in fact have the same plane of polarization, i.e. the observation made by photo detector A influenced that made by photo detector B. (See figure 22). This therefore confirms the ERP effect as predicted by quantum mechanics.

As a result Professor Lawden considers that physical systems in which psychic factors are relevant and produce changes in these systems are important areas of study. The ERP effect seems to be particularly important when considering these phenomena. Medicine testing when using BER techniques, particularly the *Vegatest* method, are just such examples of psychophysical systems displaying quantum characteristics. This is why it is of considerable importance to relate these techniques to modern scientific theory.

Professor Lawden[8] has gone on to amend the basic equations of quantum mechanics to allow for a possible disturbing psychical aspect of the system being studied and to point out certain constraints imposed on these steps by the usual assumption that quantum systems can be autonomous, i.e. independent of any influence from the consciousness of an observer. The same author finally proposes a radical transformation of quantum theory in which ideas or sensations (i.e. psychic phenomena) will provide the primary elements and the physical entities, such as atoms and radiation, will be relegated to secondary status.[9] My own view is that this may be right for the systems which show the phenomenon of collapse of the state vector on conscious observation, as described earlier, but not for other interactions (see later). Any doctor/patient interaction, even when remote such as may occur in a drug trial, is a psychophysical system where the observer effect producing collapse of the state vector and the ERP effect are important considerations.

The Experimenter (Observer) Effect
It has been known for some time that experimenters can affect the outcome of their studies. Work done by Gertrude Schmeidler in New York in the 1940s[10] showed this effect. She divided a large group of students into believers and disbelievers in ESP* (called sheep and goats respectively) and gave them a clairvoyance test using ESP cards. Not only did the sheep (believers) score significantly higher than the goats, but the latter sometimes scored significantly below chance (an unusual phenomenon). This was called a sheep/goat effect. Today the term 'sheep' is usually taken to mean

*ESP: Extra Sensory Perception.

one who believes that he can succeed in the psi test he is about to undertake, and vice versa for a 'goat'. However it has been found that some believers in ESP nevertheless consistently obtain null results (i.e. chance scoring).

The terms 'sheep' and 'goat' may refer to the experimenter or to the subject. The experimenter sheep/goat effect was demonstrated by Fisk and West in 1953.[11] They sent twenty subjects thirty-two sealed packs of clock cards (the aim was to guess the time the hour hand was pointing at), four packs at a time. Of these packs, made up in random order, sixteen had been prepared by Fisk and sixteen by West. All packs were posted by Fisk to the subjects and returned, still sealed, to him, with the subjects' guesses. The subjects were unaware that West had had any hand in the project. Furthermore, they could not have known which packs had been made up by whom. However, the scoring on Fisk's packs was highly significant (6,000 to 1 against chance) whereas on West's packs the scoring was only at chance level. The determining factor seemed to be the experimenter himself.

Rosenthal in 1963 in the USA, using a random sample of rats whose task was to learn how to escape from a maze, told his group of experimenters-to-be that half of the rats were maze 'bright' and half were maze 'dull'; he then asked them to test this experimentally. The rats then performed as the experimenters had been led to believe they would, although in fact there was no known difference between either group of rats. Several similar studies have been carried out since showing the existence of an experimenter expectancy effect.[12,13] Many workers in this field have suggested that the relationship between the subject and the experimenter is an important factor in determining whether 'sheep' would obtain higher scores than 'goats' than any direct effect of belief on scoring.

The implications for any field where psi factors are at work are therefore clear. There may be some argument as to how much of current and past medical research falls partly or wholly into this category. Perhaps this is too frightening a possibility to consider, yet it must be of crucial importance. It is certainly fundamental as far as any successful application of BER testing is concerned. The relationship of doctor and patient is crucial to its success, as suggested by the experiments mentioned above. Also the state of mind of the doctor is another important factor, again as suggested by the experimenter expectancy effect. However none of the BER techniques are totally psychokinetic phenomena, therefore some degree of objective change is also occurring, meaning that the untrained can obtain results of sorts when first starting to use these techniques. The degree of objective change varies according to the technique used, and is least in the *Vegatest* method. The equipment seems to act as a biofeedback device for the practitioner, as the performance of the tests generally improves markedly with practice, much has been found with people trained in psi tasks. This has been noted particularly by those training the military in ESP (an increasingly common practice). Those practitioners who can understand and accept the psychokinetic aspects of the *Vegatest* method of BER testing are uniformly able to translate this into becoming proficient testers. Those who cannot accept these ideas will find their results with the *Vegatest* and similar methods to be less than satisfactory.

Conclusion
It is important to recognize the part played by the practitioner in BER techniques such as the *Vegatest* method. This does not detract from their validity but merely means that the *Vegatest* and similar methods are looked at for what they are, no more and no less. They are however easier to carry out than using a totally psychic effect such as in dowsing because an objective subtle electrical change is also taking place. It may well be in the future that a method which can pick up the objective subtle electrical change alone may be developed and this is discussed in the final chapter. However this won't detract from the importance and relevance of the subjective, which the latter part of this chapter has attempted to substantiate.

7. The Theory of Homotoxicosis

One of the fundamental findings of BER medicine is that toxicity (poisoning) is a major cause of illness. These poisons have been designated homotoxins, and poisoning with them as homotoxicosis. A simple theory of the development of chronic illness due to toxins has been elaborated relying largely on ideas borrowed from naturopathy, but also on some conventional medical research. This theory is known as the theory of homotoxicosis. It cannot be recognized at the present time as being scientifically proven, but many areas of research do concur with it. It does, however, sound eminently sensible and coherent, and provides a useful framework on which to hang the hat of treatment for the clearance of toxins from the body. In this chapter, as well as explaining the theory in detail, I will also examine how good science is at assessing toxicity to chemicals. For this I have decided to look at food additives because these are a group of chemicals which most of us consume in large quantities. Lastly I will look at free oxidizing radicals as being another mechanism of action of toxins.

Natural Defences
The theory of homotoxicosis assumes that illness is the end result of a battle between homotoxins and the body's natural defences. The most important part of the body's defences lies in the immune system, which uses two main methods of dealing with invasion by foreign material: immunogobulins which are large protein molecules (known as antibodies) manufactured by special white cells against specific foreign bodies (known as antigens); and cell mediated immunity in which specialized white cells actually engulf the foreign material (known as phagocytosis) and digest it. We know a great deal about the immunoglobulin system but relatively little about cell mediated immunity. Complex homoeopathy makes

use of combinations of herbal and homoeopathic remedies which stimulate the immune system in order to facilitate the body's immune competence.

The theory of homotoxicosis claims that the autonomic nervous system (the part of the nervous system controlling unconcious internal body functions such as heart rate, intestinal muscle contraction, etc.) has a major part to play in balancing the body's natural defences between activity (stimulated by the sympathetic division of the autonomic nervous system) and quiescence (encouraged by the parasympathetic division of the autonomic nervous system). There is increasing evidence from the basic medical sciences that this may well be so. Also many of the natural therapies work through the autonomic nervous system and therefore can be expected to improve the body's natural defences.

The second arm of the body's defences lies in its methods of getting rid of toxins via three main routes of excretion: the colon, the kidneys and the skin. Methods of encouraging elimination via these routes using intestinal stimulants, diuretics (which increase urine flow) and diaphoretics (substances that increase sweating) are the corner-stone of naturopathic and herbal practice. A fundamental feature of complex homoeopathic therapy embodies these principles by including herbal preparations in complex homoeopathic mixtures to encourage elimination.

The third arm of our natural defences is the lymphatic system. This consists of a vast network of tiny capillaries which permeate all the connective tissues of the body. The lymphatics drain tissue fluid away together with toxins into large aggregations of lymphatic tissue known as lymph nodes. The toxins carried by the lymph are largely excreted into the intestinal lumen via the so-called Peyer's patches of lymphatic tissue situated just below the internal lining of the small intestine. The lymph system acts like an internal connective tissue cleansing system. Anything which impedes its flow or overwhelms it with toxins will soon give rise to a local accumulation of toxins, depending on where the problem is. Also a slight rise in pressure inside the small intestine may prejudice the fine balance which allows the lymphatics to discharge into the intestine via the Peyer's patches. Many complex homoeopathic medicaments contain effective lymphatic stimulants; this is one of the important mechanisms contributing to the effectiveness of this form of therapy. Habitual constipation can be a major problem as it predisposes to toxins remaining in the lymphatic system. We have a lot to learn from the Victorian obsession with 'bowels' and unfortunately much modern medicine has lost sight of these simple facts.

Natural history of disease due to toxins
The theory of homotoxicosis categorizes disease into three processes:

1   Toxin excretion.
2   Deposition of toxins in the tissues.
3   Tissue degeneration due to toxin deposition.

Toxins
Toxins are defined as any poisonous substances present in the body. The common toxins identified by BER medicine are listed below. They are not placed in any order of toxicity, some are clearly more toxic than others and this depends on many factors besides the toxicity of the substance itself, such as the amount present and the reaction of the tissues to it which may be more or less effective. As a rule toxins in chronic disease are not acutely poisonous but produce their effects by being present in the tissues in small amounts and continually accumulating there if exposure is continued over a long period of time. Unfortunately the body tends to store toxins in the fat cells most commonly and in various organs. Some toxins have a preference for particular organs such as the liver or the nervous system.

List of toxins
1   Industrial chemicals.
2   Pesticides, weed killers and insecticides.
3   Food additives.
4   Bacteria — often the material from the dead bodies of bacteria (which is made of protein), acts as the toxin. Live bacteria themselves are rarely toxic, but can produce chemicals which, in turn, are well recognized poisons. These chemicals, such as streptolysin produced by dividing streptococci bacteria, are usually clinically manifest during acute illness such as scarlet fever. Toxins in the sense of homotoxicosis are usually far less poisonous than substances such as streptolysin.
5   Viruses — as in bacterial toxins this usually refers to parts of the dead viral body.
6   Conventional medical drugs — especially antibiotics and mood changing drugs such as anti-depressants and anti-anxiety drugs (such as Valium).

7   Hydrocarbon based chemicals.
8   Heavy metals — such as lead and mercury. The most common
     source of mercury toxicity is from dental amalgam (the material
     out of which most dental fillings are made).

Phases of Homotoxicosis

The first phase (called the humoral phase) is one in which the toxins
are present in the extra cellular fluid. Towards the end of this phase
the toxins are beginning to move into the cells. This phase is
characterized by attempts by the body to excrete these toxins, via
the colon, urinary tract and the skin.

The second phase (known as the cellular degeneration phase)
starts with the toxins in the cells, progresses with increasing cellular
degeneration and ends with cancer. In the context of homotoxicosis
cancer is viewed as the extreme end of a degenerative process,
implying an assumed toxic cause of cancer. During the second phase
any attempts by the body to excrete toxins have no effect as the
important toxins are locked away inside the cells.

Each phase is sub-divided into three sub-phases, shown
diagrammatically below. Underneath each phase are examples from
particular diseases which clarify the concept of toxin deposition
and degeneration.

As shown on the chart, progression of disease to the right is
the natural history of increasing ill health, to the left is the natural
history of recovery. Simple measures to aid toxin excretion will
help most situations in the humoral phase (phase 1). Nosodes
(homoeopathic dilutions of toxins) are essential in the cellular
degeneration phase (phase 2). There is a very important barrier
between the two phases which is sometimes known as the biological
cesura. Once any disease is over this stage then it is much more
difficult to treat as organic cell damage is present. Therefore the
further the progression to the right the more difficult it is to institute
effective therapy. This is not so much that the toxins cannot be
removed from the cells, but that the body becomes increasingly
debilitated the more it moves to the right. This is characterized
by depletion of increasing numbers of essential enzymes, minerals
and vitamins. The emerging science of nutritional medicine has
something valuable to offer here by re-stoking the body's essential
supplies of these substances. Often the only effective way of
enabling an exhausted debilitated patient to respond to causally
directed therapy is to prescribe intensive nutritional medical therapy
specifically aimed at the deficiencies found. This sort of therapy

HUMORAL PHASE			CELLULAR DEGENERATION PHASE		
Excretion Phase	Reaction Phase	Deposition Phase	Impregnation Phase	Degeneration Phase	Neoplastic (cancerous) Phase
Characterized by the body attempting to get rid of toxins via faeces, urine, catarrh, menstrual bleeding, discharges from infected wounds, etc.	Characterized by inflammatory reactions e.g. excema, enteritis, pharyngitis, tonsillitis, appendicitis, etc	Characterized by more or less permanent cellular change due to toxin deposition, e.g. gout, benign tumours, cysts, rheumatism, etc.	Characterized by toxins being present in the cell such as liver damage (cirrhosis), various lung diseases, e.g. pneumoconiosis (due to long term exposure to coal dust) or asbestosis (due to exposure to asbestos).	Characterized by cellular degeneration due to long standing presence of toxins in the cells e.g. osteoarthritis, myocardial infarction (heart attack), emphysema.	Characterized by malignant change and the development of cancer in the tissues affected by toxins.

may have to be continued for many months before a useful improvement occurs.

Any therapy which suppresses any of the phases of homotoxicosis will encourage toxins to move intracellularly, and therefore increase the risk of chronic degenerative illness or cancer. In the sense of homotoxicosis causal treatment is based on helping the cells to excrete the toxins out into the extra-cellular fluid which bathes the cells, and from there to expel them from the system. Therefore nosode therapy and drainage remedies (see Chapter 8) are considered an essential part of treatment.

The Role of Bacteria

Bacteria are popularly regarded as being universally harmful, yet they are essential to life (see Chapter 9). It is interesting to note that most bacteria found in inflamed tissue are also found performing essential functions in the gall bladder, intestines or on the skin. The theory of homotoxicosis suggests that bacteria mop up homotoxins present in the extracellular fluid by engulfing and digesting them. In other words the bacteria perform a useful function and once the homotoxins have been removed then the bacteria will die and disappear. Furthermore the bacterial infection would not have occurred in the first place if toxins had not been present in the tissues. This implies that it is the terrain and not the bacteria which is most important. For example, one common and interesting finding is that cholera bacteria, when taken into the body, do not always cause cholera in all those who ingest them. Only those people who have the necessary toxins present, and are by implication 'under par' as far as their health is concerned, will succumb. Similar findings have been made in other bacterial and viral infections.

Other Mechanisms of Toxicity, Free Oxidizing Radicals

Oxygen is essential to life and it has an ability to react with many substances, particularly when it is present as a free oxidizing radical such as in hydrogen peroxide (H_2O_2) as opposed to water (H_2O). White blood cells produce peroxides when they attack invading bacteria in the blood or tissues. The levels of free oxidizing radicals have to be kept within certain limits otherwise they can wreak havoc by causing extensive biochemical damage to the tissues. Smog (air pollution), exhaust fumes, pesticides, insecticides and weed-killers all produce adverse effects on all of us, partly by producing an excess of free oxidizing radicals in the body. Some people respond to an excess of free oxidizing radicals with running eyes and nose, but those who get no such symptoms may well be storing up long term problems for themselves by free oxidizing radical (FOR) exposure. Foods such as coffee are also major sources. Because FORs are primarily electron donors they are particularly good at splitting double bonds and this is responsible for many of their damaging effects on the body. An important area where double bonds are essential is the double helix of DNA (deoxyribonucleic acid), out of which chromosomes are made consisting of two parallel strands of nucleotides which are held together by sulphur-sulphur double bonds. The nucleotides themselves also contain double bonds, all of which are vulnerable to oxidation and splitting by the FORs. If DNA becomes disturbed as a result of this mechanism it cannot provide correct information for cell replication, resulting in a deterioration in the efficiency of protein synthesis, with a consequent depletion of vital enzyme systems. Also disruption of the DNA may lead to abnormal cells which in some cases may develop into cancer.

All our cells contain, and are surrounded by, complex membrane systems which are made up of specialized fats called phospho-lipids. They are arranged in specific ways due to the electrical forces in their double bonds. These are particularly vulnerable to attack by FORs, which can consequently lead to cellular destruction. Luckily we have anti-oxidant systems in the body which limit the formation of FORs. These are vitamins A and E (fat-soluble vitamins), and vitamin C (water-soluble). Unfortunately the average British diet is deficient in all these vitamins, particularly vitamins A and D. Coupled with our increasing exposure to chemicals and air pollution this means that the health risks of these toxins are multiplied. Clearly a healthy nutritional approach would diminish the risks with a diet high in vegetables (especially raw vegetables as cooking destroys many essential nutrients). Surprisingly enough it is only *recently* that a major epidemiological study has been published which shows that people who have a diet high in vegetables are less at risk from cancer than those with a low vegetable intake. Clearly the FORs and the anti-oxidant vitamins A, E and C could explain this finding.

Conclusion

In the first part of this chapter I provided a model to explain the action of toxins. It must be regarded at the present time as hypotheti-cal, but whether it is capable of proof or not is another matter.

My own view is that proof isn't necessary as the theory of homotoxicosis provides workable ideas on which to hang the hat of treatment. It reinforces my feeling that ideas do not necessarily have to be correct, but they must be useful. To that extent trying to 'prove' the theory of homotoxicosis in its totality would be short sighted. There are however many separate scientific observations which support individual parts of the theory.

I then examined in a critical fashion how good science is at assessing toxicity in view of the fact that most of the substances listed as toxic in this chapter are considered, following appropriate scientific investigation, to be safe. My conclusion is that the scientific proof of toxicity is a myth and ought to be generally seen as such. We need to identify basic mechanisms by which these toxins act and attempt to monitor them. The ideas discussed in the final chapter point to possible ways of achieving this.

The last section of this chapter looks in detail at a mechanism known to science as to how some of the toxins mentioned (pesticides, weed-killers, hydrocarbon pollution, etc) produce their detrimental effects. The points made in this section are provable and point to the fact of toxicity of many everyday substances, yet we are reassured that this is not the case. A curious case of scientific double-think? From the point of view of the average man in the street it is certainly better to regard the toxins listed in this chapter as unsafe and take appropriate steps to limit exposure to them whilst maintaining optimal nutrition. The sceptic will regard all of this as unproven. Unfortunately the chances are that he will have succumbed to the toxins long before any of the quality of proven evidence he requires is on the horizon!

8. Complex Homoeopathy — A Revolution in Natural Medicine

To clarify what complex homoeopathy is, it is necessary to start with a brief résumé of the ideas behind classical homoeopathy. Homoeopathy is defined as a therapeutic method which clinically applies the law of similars and uses medically active substances at weak or infinitesimal (very diluted) doses.

The Law of Similars
The Law of Similars is the formulation of a physiological state which had already been observed by Hippocrates and his school five centuries before the birth of Christ. Even then, a similarity between the toxic power of a substance and its therapeutic action had been noted:

1 White Hellebore, which toxicologically causes cholera-like diarrhoea, was also successfully used to treat cholera.
2 Cantharide tincture, which toxicologically causes cystitis, was administered in small doses for the treatment of cystitis (at that time cystitis was known as 'strangury').

In the centuries that followed, other doctors made similar observations. They failed however to draw any practical and general conclusions. It was not until the end of the eighteenth century (around 1790) that a German doctor, chemist and toxicologist, Samuel Hahnemann, pursued the question further.

He noticed that cinchona (quinine), which was then used to treat fever resulting from malaria, toxicologically caused febrile attacks which were similar to those for which it was then used as a therapeutic remedy. Knowing as he did the works of the School of Hippocrates, he stated: 'It would appear that certain medicines are able to cure symptoms which are similar to those which they themselves can cause'. This was only a hypothesis and it needed to be verified. Hahnemann, therefore, set to work.

He began by taking all medically active substances known at that time and testing them upon himself and those around him. These substances included cinchona, aconite, belladonna, ipecacuana, mercury, etc. His goal was to find out the action of these substances upon healthy subjects. With this newly-acquired knowledge, he then tried them out as therapeutic agents upon patients showing symptoms similar to those which had been caused scientifically. He observed that his hypotheses were confirmed, but only when very small or infinitesimal doses were used. For example, when used in large quantities ipecacuana produces nausea and vomiting in the healthy individual. In small doses, it cures nausea in the dyspeptic patient. Bees' venom causes pinkish red oedema in healthy subjects. These appear suddenly and they itch and burn. They are relieved by applications of cold water. In infinitesimal doses, the same venom improves or cures itchy, burning eruptions of sudden onset and which are relieved by cold compresses.

Hahnemann thus noticed that the hypothesis he had originally formulated was regularly confirmed from one experiment to another. It was therefore no longer a hypothesis, but rather a law of nature, a general biological law, the law of similars, and could be divided into three postulates:

1   Any pharmacologically active substance can cause a set of symptoms to appear in a healthy subject. These symptoms are characteristic of each substance used. This was the result of his experiments upon healthy subjects.
2   Any one suffering from any particular disease shows a set of morbid symptoms which are characteristic of the disease. These morbid symptoms can be defined as being 'changes in the way the patient feels or behaves'.
3   The cure, which is confirmed by the objective disappearance of all morbid symptoms, may be obtained by prescribing the substance whose experimental symptoms in healthy subjects are similar to the patient's own symptoms, provided this substance is prescribed in small or infinitesimal doses. In this way, homoeopathy was born at the beginning of the nineteenth century. It had taken Hahnemann more than ten years of observations and experimentations to come to these conclusions.

As we can see from this homoeopathy is not, as some would like to believe, a crazy idea thought up by some visionary. Nor is it a philosophy or a mystical doctrine. It is rather a therapeutic method based on a hypothesis instigated by clinical facts and perfected through many years of clinical and toxicological experimentation. It consists of giving the patient, in weak or infinitesimal doses, the substance which, if administered to a healthy subject would cause symptoms similar to the patient's own symptoms. This technique might at first sight shock those used to the more direct methods related to traditional therapeutics. Indeed:

1 Classical therapeutics destroys or attempts to destroy a microbe, a virus or a parasite.
2 It chemically acts as an antidote to physiological or metabolic substances whose levels are abnormally high (uric acid, cholesterol, lipids, histamine, serotonin, etc.). It may also inhibit unpleasant or painful physiological reactions.
3 It chemically replaces inadequate physiological substances (electrolytes, hormones etc.).

Conventional therapeutics act through means involving destruction, suppression or substitution (see Chapter 4).

Homoeopathic therapeutics act in the same way as the organism's reactions. It stimulates these reactions in order to make them more effective and works in concert with them. That is the reason why only weak or even infinitesimal doses are needed: an overly strong dose could aggravate the patient's reactions in a most unpleasant way. Homoeopathic therapeutics are therefore stimulatory.

On careful consideration it is clear that conventional therapeutics often uses the law of similars:

Mercury and its salts toxicologically cause diminished urine flow or none at all. Not so long ago, mercurial diuretics (substances which cause increased urine flow) were used to treat diminished or absent urine flow of non mercurial origin.

Digitalis toxicologically causes rapid and irregular heart beats. Its best traditional indication is an irregular heart beat called auricular fibrillation wherein the heart contracts rapidly and irregularly.

Emetine toxicologically produces diarrhoea and ulcers similar to those of amoebic dysentry. Even today, it is still the best treatment when administered in doses which are far from levels which will kill the amoeba (such doses would be poisonous to man). Emetine acts by stimulating the organism's natural defences.

Small-pox vaccination also illustrates the law of similars. When the 'vaccine' is inoculated it produces skin sores similar to those of smallpox.

It is possible to quote many more examples, especially in allergy or in immunology, where small doses of the same substances capable of producing pathological disorders are used as therapeutic agents. There is nothing surprising about this. The law of similars is a general biological law and it is normal for traditional therapeutics to use it. The only difference is that the homoeopathic therapist uses it systematically.

Pathogenesis
The set of symptoms which any given substance produces in a healthy individual is called pathogenesis. These symptoms come mainly from three sources:

Toxicology — this may be acute, chronic, voluntary, accidental or professional. It usually causes physical damage.

Actual pathogenetic experiments — these are carried out with diverse but non-poisonous agents upon subjects of various ages, of both sexes, and of different receptivity. They mainly cause functional or general signs, in other words 'changes in the way of feeling or behaving' (Hahnemann).

Clinical experiments — these include symptoms which are normally cured by the prescribed substance in its pathogenesis.

The homoeopathic Materia Medica
The total sum of these pathogeneses constitute the homoeopathic *Materia Medica*. The *Materia Medica* is a collection of symptoms, 'changes in the way of feeling or behaving' in healthy individuals. These symptoms are of local, general, functional and behavioural nature. They are produced by pharmacologically active substances.

Methodology in Homoeopathy
Knowing, as he does, the homoeopathic *Materia Medica*, the homoeopathic doctor must take into account the symptoms of the patient within his disease; in other words, the way he reacts to it. The doctor will therefore prescribe the substance whose experimental reactional modalities correspond to those of the patient. The remedy is 'homoeopathic' because its basic substance is capable of creating a 'similar' (homoeo = similar) 'suffering' (pathos = suffering).

Let us examine one case in point: two patients suffering from shingles who both consult the doctor. The first patient has a rash; he suffers from itching, burning pains. These pains are relieved by cold compresses. This reaction is exactly the same as that of a healthy person who has been stung by a bee. The homoeopathic remedy will therefore be bee venom in an infinitesimal dilution. The second patient also has a rash and complains of burning pains. Questioning, however, reveals that the patient's pains are worse at night and that they are relieved by hot compresses. This patient's reaction is therefore completely different from that of the first patient even though the disease is the same. This reaction corresponds to that of a healthy individual subjected to the toxicological action of arsenious anhydride in an infinitesimal dilution.

Homoeopathic methodology then, consists of making two symptomatic clinical pictures coincide in order to determine the remedy or remedies to be used. The first of these clinical pictures is that concerning the pathogenesis. This is the reactive picture of a healthy individual undergoing the action of a pharmacologically active substance. The second is the patient's symptomatic clinical picture. This includes both the characteristic sign of the disease and particular signs shown in the patient's behaviour. It is the picture of the patient's reaction to his illness.

Homoeopathic methodology thus leads to an individualization of therapy. It defines the remedy which works in the same direction as the patient's own reaction which it helps and stimulates. Homoeopathic therapeutics involve individual terrains. Homoeopathic remedies act as a specific stimulant to the organism as opposed to traditional remedies which act coercively.

The Infinitesimal Dose

In order to spare the patient from unpleasant reactions due to the worsening of his condition, this stimulation must not be too strong. It must act only as a support or an encouragement to the organism. It was only after years of experiment that Hahnemann came to the following conclusion: 'in order to bring about prompt, gentle, and lasting improvement, you most often need to use infinitesimal doses'. Hahnemann himself codified the preparation of these doses.

Because these doses are infinitesimal, homoeopathic medicine is never poisonous. The only problem is to define how it works as, in itself, it has no chemical action. It acts exclusively through a specific physical state which is capable of making only the affected organism react because it is sensitized to the medicine through its own specific reactive mode (which is itself similar to the reactive potential of the basic substance). This will be discussed in more detail in a later section. To illustrate this process better, we might liken the organism to a radio receiver which is capable of receiving and amplifying only those waves into which it is tuned.

HOMOEOPATHIC MEDICATIONS

Origin

Homoeopathy is often wrongly identified as herbal therapy. Homoeopathic remedies are prepared from substances belonging to all three realms of nature:

The vegetable kingdom — this kingdom is the source of more than half the remedies. Plants are harvested in their natural surroundings by qualified specialists who obey strict quality standards. They are then quickly dispatched to the laboratory so they can be used fresh (having first been subjected to a thorough botanical check-up).

The mineral kingdom — this includes natural salts, chemical products, metals, etc. They are always selected in their purest state.

The animal kingdom — these substance includes venoms, venomous insects (bees, ants, spiders, etc.), hormones, physiological secretions (musk, squid ink, etc.), and any substance capable of having a toxicological or pharmacodynamic action upon a healthy individual.

Preparation

Preparation is given very careful attention. Vegetable substances as well as some animal substances are used to prepare Mother Tinctures (M.T.). This is carried out by maceration in alcohol for at least three weeks. Maceration takes place either in specially treated glass vessels or in stainless-steel containers. A very pure alcohol is used. This alcohol is exactly titrated. Mother Tinctures are concentrated in such a way that their weight is equal to ten times that of the dried plant and twenty times that of animal products.

Mother Tinctures and soluble products are the basic substances which are then diluted to 1/10th or 1/100th part. At each stage of deconcentration the medicine undergoes energetic shaking by a machine called a 'potentizer'. It is then labelled with the Latin name of the stock used, followed by a number representing the number of deconcentrations and shakings which it has undergone, and an acronym indicating whether the deconcentration was to the 1/10th or to the 1/100th:

6X or 6D means that the basic substance has been deconcentrated to the 1/10 part, 6 times and then shaken 6 times. The dilution therefore contains one part in a million.

5C means that the basic substance has been deconcentrated to the 1/100 part, 5 times and then shaken 5 times. The dilution contains one part in ten billion.

Deconcentrations which are potentized in this way are called Hahnemannian potencies.

Insoluble basic substances are divided three times to the 1/100th by trituration with lactose in a mortar. Research, for which a Doctor of Science Degree was awarded, showed that when an insoluble substance was triturated to the 3C and beyond, it could be deconcentrated by diluting it in the same way as a soluble product.

The most frequently used dilutions in homoeopathic remedies are:

M.T. — 3X 6X 4C 5C 7C 9C 12C 15C 30C

Nowadays, the manufacture of Hahnemannian potencies (dilutions) necessitates special precautions. It is, of course, important to use very pure solvents: 70 per cent strength alcohol and distilled water. It is also preferable to carry out the preparation of these potencies (dilutions) in the purest possible atmosphere. It is hardly necessary to state that the normal atmosphere is polluted. It contains a great number of particles (chemical or otherwise) which are in suspension and which can be detected and counted with special equipment. The presence of sulphur, calcium, sodium, potassium, sulphurous or arsenious anhydride, lead, mercury, and many other poisonous or allergenic products can be shown. These elements all contribute to pollution. These substances exist in concentrations which are higher than those of the homoeopathic remedies being made and they could easily be solubilized and potentized during the preparation of successive dilutions.

In Hahnemann's day, atmospheric pollution was negligible when the first pathogeneses were established and the first homoeopathic medicines made, air pollution was not a problem. Nowadays, however, it is a real obstacle. These polluting substances could, under certain circumstances, overpower the active ingredients if insufficient precautions were taken during manufacture.

Complex Homoeopathy

Complex homoeopathy is a method of formulating medications which was initially developed by one of Hahnemann's pupils. It involves the use of mixtures of Mother Tinctures and low potency homoeopathic preparations (usually between 6C and 12C). These mixtures are formulated so as to minimize any aggravation that might be caused by the homoeopathic preparations and to maximize the effect of that preparation on a particular organ, or for a particular symptom. They combine the best features of homoeopathy and herbal medicine. Classical homoeopathy misses out on the age-old methods of drainage via the colon, urinary tract and skin. Complex homoeopathy combines these approaches together with the ideas of homoeopathy.

The importance of using a number of remedies rather than the classical similimum, is shown by all the BER techniques. Invariably the majority of patients need a number of remedies in order to normalize all abnormal readings. It is important that all remedies given together are compatible with each other. Compatibility testing both clinically and using BER testing is an important step at arriving at the formulations used in complex homoeopathy.

The resultant mixtures are found to act on particular organs or organ systems; some stimulate the pancreas or liver, others aid the circulation or facilitate lymphatic drainage. It is therefore a therapeutic system ideally suited to the organ-based diagnoses made in BER medicine. Some complex homoeopathic mixtures are targeted at conditions such as sinusitis or tonsillitis. They are easy to use, even for the layman and are used in this way by many people today in Germany where the majority of complex homoeopathic medications are made.

In my experience the clinical results from the use of complex homoeopathy in chronic disease are better than when using classical single remedy homoeopathy on the same cases. As far as acute illness is concerned there is little difference between the two systems, and both methods are fairly simple to apply in the acute situation (such as the use of *Belladonna 6C*, a classical single remedy in tonsillitis, or the use of *Mercurius Cyanatus*, a complex remedy for the same problem). Chronic illness is a much more complex problem and needs much greater skill and experience in classical homoeopathy for the treatment to be successful. In practice very few homoeopaths have this sort of skill, but they do obtain a proportion of dramatic results. From my own observation the proportion of significant results in chronic illness using single remedy classical homoeopathy is as low as 45 per cent. My experience with complex homoeopathy reveals that approximately 75 per cent of patients can be helped. Clearly the complex approach has the edge as far as results are concerned, and when used in tandem with BER diagnosis, provides a system much more related to conventional medicine than is classical homoeopathy.

Unfortunately the argument between the 'singles' and the 'complex' schools rages, with relatively few open-minded practitioners recognizing that both have a part to play. Experience with measurement techniques used in BER medicine shows that the complex approach turns out to be the most favoured method; and that classical homoeopathy with its reliance on symptom pictures is by implication out-dated.

The use of complex or mixed homoeopathic preparations is common in many European countries, particularly Germany. As yet this approach has not been widely used in the United Kingdom or the USA. Complex homoeopathic preparations involve relatively low potency medications and are mixtures of several different medicaments. For instance *Belladonna* (made by Pascoe Pharmaceuticals in West Germany) contains *Belladonna, Bryonia* and *Mercurius Sublimatus.* All of these are in low potency, and the addition of Bryonia and Mercurius Sublimatus, is to avoid and minimize the occurrence of side effects that may occur by prescribing *Belladonna* alone. A complex preparation also has a wider range of action than a single remedy. This means that it is more likely to produce a clinically useful result. In other words a mixed complex remedy is a balanced herbal and homoeopathic combination preparation which aims to achieve its effect with minimum possible disruption to the patient.

As a rule each complex homoeopathic preparation has been given a trade name by the pharmacy producing it. Often this trade name is that of the classical single remedy such as, in this case, *Belladonna.* It is important to realize that this isn't the same thing as the classical single remedy *Belladonna.*

Nosodes
Nosodes are homoeopathic dilutions of toxins (see Chapter 7). Their effect is to cause the body to expel the toxins relevant to the particular nosode from an intra-cellular position into the extra-cellular fluid. It is a remarkable fact that a homoeopathic dilution of a toxin will specifically stimulate the cells to discharge the relevant toxin into the extra-cellular fluid. This effect has been extensively researched and a number of representative studies will be described in the following section.

At best nosodes should be given only after using a measurement technique on the patient such as the *Vegatest* method so that the right preparation is chosen. Nosodes should never be given alone, and should always be given with the relevant accompanying remedies whose function is to make sure that the toxins, now in the extra-cellular fluid, are excreted from the body. If this is not done then the toxins will remain in the extra-cellular fluid for a while and then go back into the cells. This has been called 'toxic ping-pong', and underlines the need to give drainage remedies at the same time. This is another area where complex homoeopathy has a real edge over classical homoeopathy, as it makes extensive use of drainage remedies of various sorts.

Nosodes should not be used for self-treatment, and should always be given under the guidance of an appropriately trained practitioner. They should not be given to the very elderly or frail patients, as the sudden release of toxins into the extra-cellular fluid may be more than the patient can cope with.

Bach Flower Remedies

These are a group of thirty-eight remedies made from common flowers such as Clematis, Vervain and Star of Bethlehem. They were 'invented' by Dr Edward Bach, working in the 1930s. They all have an effect on the psychological aspects of a patient's problem, and to that end they are invaluable. High potency single remedy prescribing also has dramatic effects on the psyche but requires far greater knowledge and clinical experience to be able to use high potency single remedy prescribing safely and effectively. Only skilled and experienced homoeopathic practitioners are competent at this approach. The Bach remedies are, however, safe, and they can be used for self-treatment. In my view they are an essential part of the therapeutic range required by BER medicine. Bach remedies have the effect of bringing problems to the surface, and therefore making them more amenable to resolution. If a patient has a more deep-seated psychological problem then no homoeopathic remedy will resolve it, and a psychologically based method of treatment is required.

Research Evidence for the Activity of Substances at Infinitesimal Doses

Even though homoeopathy was founded upon strict observation and experiment, it has always been the object of criticism. Homoeopaths have always tried to provide an answer to this criticism. It is only in the last forty years, however, that research techniques have improved to such a point that scientific proof can be shown as a reply to the various objections.

Rather than involving ourselves in a history of the research into homoeopathy including an exhaustive analysis of all the experiments carried out by chemists, pharmacologists, doctors, engineers, and physicists (many of whom are professors of medicine and pharmacy), let us instead say that research has tried to demonstrate:

1   That the pharmacological action of Hahnemannian potencies could be shown by reproducible and statistically valid procedures.
2   That, because the activity of these potencies was connected to a specific physical structure, they consequently were not just empty solutions or 'solutions with nothing in them' as they have often been called.
3   That homoeopathic therapeutics do not act by auto-suggestion or placebo effect.

It should be stressed that research in the homoeopathic field is essentially fundamental research. It thus differs from the type of research usually carried out in clinical pharmacology where the goal is to show the therapeutic action of a new product.

Pharmacological Action of Hahnemannian Potencies
Faced with the impossible task of causing a direct pharmacological action in healthy subjects, researchers had the idea of experimenting with the pharmacological action of homoeopathic medicines upon 'sensitized' animals or plants. Thus:

1   If pigeons are poisoned with sodium arsenate, only 35 per cent of the poison administered will be found in their excreta in the days following the experiment. At the same time, there is an increase in vestibular chronaxia showing precisely this sub-intoxication (vestibular = the balance apparatus; chronaxia = time taken for nerve conductions).
     If the pigeons are than given Hahnemannian potencies of sodium arsenate at 7C, 9C or 15C strength about forty-five days after the initial poisoning, arsenic reappears in the excreta and vestibular chronaxia returns to normal in a few days.
2   If Alloxan is given to mice, it produces experimental diabetes (increase in blood sugar), by destroying certain pancreatic cells. If the mice are given preventive injections of infinitesimal potencies of Alloxan, they do not develop diabetes. If infinitesimal potencies are injected for a few days following the injection of Alloxan, both the diabetes and pancreatic lesions produced are much less serious.
3   If grains of wheat are poisoned with copper sulphate, their

'vitality' is considerably modified, especially their germination potential: the weight of roots and coleoptiles, chlorophyl production and enzyme activities are greatly reduced in comparison to normal grains. If, however, these poisoned grains are planted in soil to which a 15C potency of copper sulphate has been added, all of these parameters are significantly improved and come near to those of healthy grains.

4   A trial looking at the effect of homoeopathic lead as a method for lowering lead levels in experimental adult rats was reported at the 35th Congress of the International Homoeopathic Medical League at the University of Sussex, Brighton, in March 1982, the work having been carried out by Dr Peter Fisher. The rats were divided into four groups. One group received homoeopathic treatment of *Plumbum Metallicum 200C* (homoeopathic lead), the second group received *Penicillamine* (a standard method for reducing toxic metals in the body), and the third group were an alcohol treated control group as the *Plumbum Metallicum 200C* was given in absolute alcohol diluted with distilled water. The fourth group was another control group treated with water alone. The results showed that *Plumbum Metallicum 200C* was better at producing lead excretion than *Penicillamine,* although the difference was only slight. The difference between lead excretion between the *Plumbum Metallicum 200C* and the *Penicillamine* group compared to the water and alcohol control groups was shown to be highly significant, and in both control groups there was negligible excretion of lead.

5   If rats are injected with carbon or phosphorous tetrachloride, toxic liver damage is caused. If, after poisoning rats with carbon tetracholoride, they are given injections of 7C or 15C potencies of phosphorus, their hepatitis improves as well as their abnormal biochemical parameters (especially transaminases), which return to normal.

These experiments show the action of infinitesimal dilutions, even those in which it is not possible to find molecules of the basic substances (greater than Avogadro's number) still present in these dilutions.

A study of the physical structure of Hahnemannian potencies
When a substance is diluted in a solvent, several complex phenomena are brought into play:

1   The dispersion of molecules: the physical difference between

one gram of sodium chloride in a solid form, and one gram of the same substance dissolved in 1, 10 or 100 litres of water is clear. The relative arrangement of the molecules is not the same.

It is just as clear as the difference existing between the molecular arrangement of water molecules (H-OH) in a liquid state, a solid state (ice) or a gaseous state (steam).

Even though the chemical formula is unchanged in both these examples, the physical constants, as well as their possible areas of application are not the same.

When making dilutions, however, the dispersion of molecules of the substances to be diluted amongst those of the solvent is not the only factor involved. There is also:

2   A specific molecular arrangement between the two components. For example, in an aqueous dilution, each molecule or ion of the diluted substance is surrounded by water molecules. This makes a hydrated molecule or ion with completely new properties.

When another dilution is made, this molecular arrangement varies, not only for each molecule of the basic substance, but also in relation to the substance.

It follows, then, that each time a product is diluted in a solvent, a new physico-chemical entity is created. Its properties are not only proportional to the quantities of substance used. To illustrate this idea, let us say that, when one blue marble is mixed with 99 yellow marbles, the result is 100 green marbles with new and not always predictable properties.

It is thus reasonable to imagine that comparable phenomena take place in Hahnemannian potencies, and that they are helped along by the way of preparing these successive dilutions.

If the Hahnemannian dilution is submitted to ultrasound or to heat (20 minutes at 120°C), the dilution's pharmacological power is destroyed. Furthermore, when these potencies are subjected to a laser beam (monochromatic luminous beam) and the different diffusions produced are recorded on a Raman spectrograph, specific spectra are obtained. This very delicate research seems to show certain differences between the spectra of the solvent and those of the various dilutions studied.

There is, therefore, every reason to think that this specific physical state carries the reactional and therapeutical potential of a substance diluted in accordance with the Hahnemannian procedure.

The Placebo Effect

It would be childish to try to deny the existence of the placebo effect for it can be found in all kinds of therapeutics. The moment the patient consults a doctor, a relationship is created between the two parties, and this can more or less calm the patient's fears. This is just as true for homoeopathy as for classical medicine. Care must be taken when interpreting therapeutic results. A treatment can be prescribed (whatever that treatment may be) just as much for the feeling of security it gives the patient as for its actual pharmacological action.

Therapeutic results obtained by homoeopathy in functional disorders, dystonias, and anxiety, therefore, do not constitute scientific proof of the action of the homoeopathic remedy — many other factors could be responsible for the improvement. This same scepticism is no longer justified however, when the following are concerned:

- cure of infectious diseases;
- focal disorders;
- normalizing serum measurements;
- cures brought about in babies or in young children;
- cures in isolated animals or in herds (veterinary medicine increasingly uses homoeopathy both for pets, farm animals, and race horses).

Even in the above cases, however, these cures are not scientific evidence of activity. A scientific phenomenon is recognized as such only when it has been proved to be statistically significant and reproducible.

After reading this highly simplified account the reader will realize that homoeopathy is a therapeutic method that deserves to be both better known and more widely used. It does not replace classical medicine, but it can often be a useful addition to it.

Conclusion

Complex homoeopathy has in many ways updated classical homoeopathy and certainly has made it an easier therapeutic system to apply in practice. Research in homoeopathy has also reached a level where we can begin to say that real effects are produced by these sorts of remedies.

9. Dysbiosis — An Unrecognized Epidemic

Dysbiosis, sometimes called dysbacteria, is a condition in which abnormal intestinal bacteria are present. It is exceptionally common and is largely unrecognized by conventional medicine. The normal bowel bacteria (known as bacterial flora) are 95 per cent anaerobic (this means that they do not use oxygen and are killed by contact with oxygen). They mainly consist of the following types: bacteroides, bacterium bifidum, various strains of escherichia coli, enterococci and lactobacilli. Proteus, yeasts, clostridia, staphyloccocci and aerobic spore producers are found in small numbers. These organisms form a symbiotic relationship (a biological relationship in which both host and bacteria benefit) with the colon, and the consequence of their absence has been clearly demonstrated by experiments with animals reared in germ-free environments. These animals soon succumb to fatal infection when released into the normal environment.

Symptom Complex of Dysbiosis
Symptoms are usually intestinal, such as flatulence, disordered bowel habit and intermittent abdominal swelling. Hypotheses on the subject of dysbiosis are legion and unfortunately often contradictory. Dysbiosis covers the symptom complexes of irritable bowel syndrome, spastic colon, ulcerative colitis and some cases of Crohn's disease. The concept of dysbiosis seems to be a peculiarly German one, but for all that it is an eminently practical approach to an exceptionally common problem.

Relationships of the Bacterial Flora
There appears to be a physiological symbiotic balance between the acidophilus-bifidum group of bacteria and the coliform organisms (escherichia coli). If the coliform bacteria predominate

then there is a tendency for the flora to rise in the intestine towards the small intestine. If the acidophilus – bifidum group (which are known as lactic acid fermenters) predominate, then the coliform bacteria are no longer able to function properly as the optimal colonic pH (a measure of the acidity/alkalinity), which must be slightly alkaline, is changed because of the excess acid production of the lactic acid fermentor organisms. It should therefore be possible to treat dysbiosis with either preparations of coliform organisms or of the acidophilus organisms.

Most importantly there appears to be a relationship between the permeability (a measure of the ability to filter substances through) of the gut mucous membrane (the internal gut lining) and normal bowel flora. If the flora is abnormal or unbalanced then the gastro-intestinal mucous membrane becomes abnormally permeable, rather like a sieve in which the holes are too big, allowing the absorption of inadequately broken down proteins and the reabsorption of toxins from the bowel contents. This is often what happens in food sensitivity, and in my experience dysbiosis is a major underlying cause of such sensitivity.[1] Simply treating the dysbiosis results in the eventual disappearance of the majority of food sensitivities in patients who are allergic to a variety of foods.

The toxins and proteins absorbed from the gut enter the liver circulation (known as the portal circulation) and may produce pharmacological effects due to the proteins or toxic effects due to the reabsorbed toxins. This may go some way towards explaining why the simultaneous administration of a liver remedy is essential when treating dysbiosis.

Causes of Dysbiosis
Dysbiosis has many causes, of which the most important will be discussed here. The most common is antibiotic usage. Antibiotics tend to be used in a cavalier fashion and as a result very few of us have not had at least one course of antibiotics, probably unnecessarily in most cases. As a result the colonic flora is permanently damaged in many people. A proportion regain their normal bacteria, especially if they are sensible enough to take plenty of live yogurt (which contains acidophilus bacteria) following a course of antibiotics. Widespread antibiotic usage is probably the most important cause of dysbiosis at the present time. Unfortunately doctors are not the only ones who use antibiotics. Veterinary surgeons do as well, with the consequence that many animal carcasses are contaminated with antibiotic residues, which are

ultimately eaten with the meat. The only way of avoiding this is to become a vegetarian (as I have done) or eat meat reared in the wild such as venison or game.

Other factors which cause dysbiosis are poor nutrition, particularly the consumption of large quantities of junk food; also any severe illness which causes a consequent rush of toxins which are discharged from the body via the colon, which can upset the flora. Clearly any enteritis, especially if infective, will also by its very nature upset the normal bacterial population.

Functional and organic disease of the gastro-intestinal tract together with dysfunction of the liver and pancreas commonly go hand in hand with dysbiosis, which should therefore be looked for in cases of gastritis, hepatitis or pancreatitis. Pancreatic or liver dysfunction will upset the gastro-intestinal pH (the acid/alkaline level) which is critical for the gut flora to function normally. For example, if the stomach produces too much acid (as in hyperacidic gastritis) then the alkaline bile, pancreatic and small intestine secretions are not sufficient to neutralize the excess gastric acid. As a result digestion is incomplete and becomes subject to fermentation processes if there is excess carbohydrate intake. In these situations there will be excessive gas production and abdominal distension. If protein forms a large part of the diet then there will be putrefaction with foul smelling intestinal gas. In both cases an excessive bacterial colonization of the bowel occurs with a consequently increased fermentation or putrefaction depending on whether the diet predominates in carbohydrates or proteins, which in the end will produce a dysbacteria.

Stress, that ubiquitous cause of many illnesses, affects the gastro-intestinal lining membrane which can in turn cause changes in the normal gut flora leading to an invasion of bacteria foreign to the intestine.

Normal functions of the bowel flora
Bowel bacteria are essential to the development of a normal immune system, as experiments with germ-free animals has shown. In these animals the weight and length of the small intestine, for example, is reduced as is the lymphatic system.

Intestinal bacteria can synthesize vitamins, mostly of the B group, but also vitamin K. In dysbiosis the majority of vitamins taken by mouth, either in the food or by vitamin replacements, will be taken up by the abnormal bacteria, resulting in vitamin deficiency. This may well be why large doses of vitamins are found to be effective, whereas low doses often produce no result. Orthomolecular medicine, which has as its hallmark the administration of megadoses of vitamins and minerals, has been based on this observation. My suggestion is that if the underlying dysbiosis was adequately treated then smaller doses of vitamins would be adequate.

The Candida problem
Within the discipline of clinical ecology candida sensitivity is considered to be of major importance, [2] and its recognition is often fundamental to the successful resolution of multiple food sensitivities in many patients. In my experience if the dysbiosis is resolved successfully using complex homoeopathy and appropriate supporting measures, then the candida problem, which is secondary to this, will then disappear with most, if not all, of the food sensitivities.

Diseases in which dysbiosis is commonly found as a main or contributing cause
Dysbiosis could be regarded as a 'basic illness' with many symptoms. As well as the obvious bowel problems already mentioned, such as ulcerative colitis or diverticulitis, the following illnesses, apparently bearing no relation whatsoever to the colon, are regularly helped significantly by the identification and treatment of an underlying dysbiosis:

- Liver, gall bladder and pancreatic dysfunction
- Acne
- Fungal infections such as candida
- Asthma
- Urticaria
- Eczema
- Post-viral debility
- Rheumatism

The Diagnosis of Dysbiosis
The history is the most important pointer, but will not be obvious when dysbiosis is present as a hidden underlying cause of the diseases mentioned in the previous section. Constipation, flatulence, morning diarrhoea or any irregular bowel habit, foul smelling faeces, and intermittent abdominal swelling all point to a possible dysbiosis.

The diagnosis can also be made by bacteriological examination of the faeces. In practice this is a laborious and expensive procedure due to the fact that most bowel organisms are anaerobic, and so have to be grown in special cabinets from which the air has been excluded.

BER techniques provide the best methods of diagnosis either using the *Segmental Electrogram* or the *Vegatest* method, or both.

The Treatment of Dysbiosis

The mainstays of treatment are replacing the normal flora by using live preparations of bacteria and stimulating the associated organs of the gastro-intestinal tract, such as the liver and the pancreas.

The treatment falls into three stages depending on the severity of the dysbiosis. In all cases obvious primary causes (such as psychological stress) must be identified and dealt with adequately, and also appropriate nosodes, if indicated, need to be given. The *Vegatest* method is the best way of determining this.

In all cases the diagnosis in terms of stressed organs and testing of the prescription for effectiveness and suitability should be carried out using a BER technique. In this section complex homoeopathic preparations made mostly by Pascoe Pharmaceuticals Limited will be mentioned. However, there is no good evidence to suggest that the complex homoeopathic preparations made by one pharmacy are any better than those produced by another, the secret of success is correct diagnosis and a judicious combination of remedies chosen to fit this. The addresses of other complex homoeopathic pharmacies are appended at the end of this book.

Stage 1 (the average case)
A combination of remedies for disorders of the large intestine, liver and pancreas will sort out most of these cases. Occasionally a nosode is also needed. The large intestine remedies I use with regularity are the following:

> *Markalakt* powder (Pascoe Pharmacy)
> *Dysbiosan* tablets (Pascoe Pharmacy)
> *Hylac Forte* drops (Merckle Pharmacy)

Liver Preparations:

> *Lycopodium* drops — this is the best tolerated but least powerful
>   liver remedy (Pascoe Pharmacy)

Hepar Pasc tablets (Pascoe Pharmacy)
Liver Meridian Complex No. 7 (Kern Pharmacy)
Legapas drops — this is the strongest liver remedy (Pascoe Pharmacy)

Pancreatic Preparations:

Phaseolus drops — this is the best tolerated pancreatic remedy (Pascoe Pharmacy)
Pascopancreat drops — this is the strongest and most effective pancreatic remedy (Pascoe Pharmacy)

Gastric Preparations:

For acidic gastritis:
Nux Vomica or *Artemesia Similiaplexe* (Pascoe Pharmacy)
For hypo-acidic gastritis:
Thymus Similiaplexe or *Amara* drops (Pascoe Pharmacy)

Stage II (more severe cases)
In these cases a simultaneous dietary approach must also be considered. Additional therapy to Stage I consists of giving live bacterial preparations to re-seed the colon with normal bowel flora. A number of courses may need to be given as at least 70 per cent of the bacteria taken by mouth will be destroyed by the gastric acid. Multivitamin therapy in high doses can also be added in these cases.

List of preparations containing live bacteria:

Hylac Forte — this contains Lactobacillus acidophillus, Strepotococcus faecalis and Escheria coli (Merckle Pharmacy)
Omniflora — containing Lactobacillus acidophillus, Lactobacillus bifidum and Escheria coli (MED Fabrik Pharmacy)
Symbioflor I and II — containing Strepotococcus faecalis and Escheria coli (Mikrobiologische Laboratories)
Eugalan Topfer Forte — containing bacterium bifidum (made by Topfer Pharmacy)

Eugalan Topfer Forte is the treatment of choice in dysbiosis in children because of their different (normal) bowel flora to adults.

It is also of proven use in liver failure (emphasizing the functional connection between the liver and the colon).

Stage II (the most severe cases)
These patients often need a series of high colonic wash-outs to remove all putrefied and hardened post-putrefactive material from the colon. Replacement of normal bowel flora as detailed in Stage II needs to be given following the wash-outs as the bacteria are often removed following such treatment.

Therapy as detailed in Stages I and II needs to be given. In some cases antibiotics ought to be considered to remove the abnormal bacteria present, but these must only be given under adequate medical supervision.

Dietary Regime in Cases of Dysbiosis

Some foods cause mucous secretion which in turn causes the stools to become sticky. This lengthens transit time and so predisposes to the accumulation of putrefying material in the colon, thereby blocking lymphatic drainage of toxins from Peyer's patches into the bowel lumen. Avoidance of these foods and the addition of vegetable roughage can pay enormous dividends to many patients, as well as those with dysbiosis.

Foods to be avoided:
   Meat, particularly red meat
   Milk and dairy products, including goats milk
   Eggs
   Soya
   Processed foods.

The diet should consist of:
Vegetables in quantity, particularly raw carrots, cauliflower and cabbage. This is an important source of vegetable roughage and is less irritant to the colon than wheat bran. Fruit in quantity, grains, nuts, beans, legumes. This diet is a low-fat vegetarian diet. It is also the diet recommended for patients with malignancy.

Many people reading this chapter will recognize various symptoms which would suggest that dysbiosis is their problem. A simple application of the dietary measures together with some of the homoeopathic preparations mentioned will be adequate to sort out most of these simple problems.

10. Common Disease States Shown by Bio-electronic Regulatory Medicine

A number of common disease states are revealed by bio-electronic regulatory techniques. These are geopathic stress, chronic sinusitis, chronic tonsillitis, chronic appendicitis, dental foci, salmonella toxicity, streptococcal toxicity and post-viral states. I will describe each of these briefly, as they are relatively common and important clinical problems.

Geopathic Stress
This has been described on page 62. I have been impressed with the finding that patients with geopathic stress tend not to respond to any therapy which involves an energetic approach such as acupuncture or homoeopathy. Once the geopathic stress has been corrected, then the patient often begins to respond. Nevertheless it remains a difficult area as, with present technology, it is impossible to define precisely the presumed abnormalities in the geomagnetic field in which the patient is living. Patients are much more likely to be affected by geopathic stress in the place in which they sleep. During the daytime when the sympathetic division of the autonomic nervous system is dominant, and as a consequence the body's energy field seems to be larger, then it appears easier for people to withstand any geopathic stress which may happen to be present. Geopathic stress certainly does not affect everybody living in a particular environment; only those individuals who are sufficiently sensitive respond to these subtle changes.

Chronic Sinusitis
Chronic sinusitis is a common and often unrecognized problem. Conventional diagnosis relies on the patient's history and X-ray examination. BER techniques, however, show that chronic sinusitis is present in many patients whose sinus X-rays are normal.

The eight sinuses are situated in the head and are paired. They are the maxillary, frontal, ethmoid and sphenoidal sinuses. The maxillary sinus, situated on each side of the nose just behind the cheeks, is related to the stomach meridian, the frontal sinus to the bladder meridian and the ethmoid cells immediately on each side of the nose, to the large intestine meridian. The sinuses appear to act as 'vents' for these organs. The implication is that sinusitis is nearly always secondary to something going on elsewhere in the body, most commonly in the large intestine, stomach or bladder. This is because of the meridian connections of these sinuses as detailed above. For example, it often turns out that stress of the large intestine (dysbiosis) turns out to be the underlying cause for many cases of chronic sinusitis. Treating the dysbiosis often precipitates copious secretion from the sinuses as the body attempts to resolve the situation.

Treatment of chronic sinusitis
Local measures such as sinus wash-outs can be used and indeed are routine in conventional medicine. Antibiotics are commonly used within conventional medicine when an infection is present. This often relieves the uncomfortable pressure which acute sinusitis can bring. However, in the long run this does not produce any long-term improvement, and if there is an underlying dysbiosis repeated courses of antibiotics will make the bacterial situation in the intestine even worse.

Complex Homoeopathy should be directed at the sinusitis using, for example, *Kalium Chloratum* (Pascoe Pharmacy) and also at the underlying problem such as dysbiosis.

Chronic Tonsillitis
The tonsillar ring of lymphatic tissue often acts as a secondary focus (a focus is defined as the presence of non-absorbable material in the connective tissue). The focal effect of the tonsils can continue after surgical removal due to scar tissue formation and consequent blocking of the local lymphatics, preventing the complete removal of pus and dead tissue. Therefore in some instances, due to poorly executed surgery, the tonsils can be converted from a secondary to a primary focus. The tonsils can be important starting points for rheumatic fever and the rheumatic group of diseases. This is accepted conventional teaching. BER techniques and complex homoeopathy provide a way to treat these chronic diseases by directing therapy at the long-standing tonsillar foci.

The primary factors responsible for 'activating' the tonsils are due to their meridian relationships. These are most commonly the large intestine followed by the liver and the endocrine meridians (the so-called triple warmer meridians in traditional Chinese medicine), and all these pass through the tonsils. Some patients being treated for their liver or colon often develop a sore throat during treatment, therefore confirming this relationship. As for sinusitis treatment is directed locally by using, for example, *Mercurius Cyanatus* drops (Pascoe Pharmacy) and also towards the underlying cause given by the meridian relationship of the tonsils which may be the large intestine (i.e. dysbiosis) or the liver or endocrine system.

Chronic Appendicitis
Chronic appendicitis is an under-diagnosed but important primary focus which can be responsible for a wide range of different conditions such as irritable bowel syndrome, rheumatoid arthritis or multiple food and chemical sensitivity, to name a few. Clinical examination, investigation and history are all unrealiable indicators to this diagnosis. BER techniques are the diagnostic methods of choice.

The *Segmental Electrogram* can give some indication as to whether complex homoeopathy is likely to be successful or not in resolving a chronic appendix or whether surgery will be required. If the recording post-stimulation on the *SEG* becomes larger in all the quadrants then it is likely that conservative therapy will be successful (i.e. complex homoeopathy). If the post-stimulation recording shows smaller deflections than the pre-stimulation one then this indicates so-called negative regulation which means that surgery would almost certainly be required. To date I have gathered a series of twelve cases with chronic appendicitis all diagnosed using BER techniques. All twelve were operated on and ten of them had abnormal appendices when examined under the microscope. Nine out of the twelve started to respond to therapy once the appendix had been removed. Three cases showed no change. The appendix therefore was acting like any primary focus in that it was preventing the patient responding usefully to conservative therapy.

Dental Foci
Dental foci, in common with other foci, are usually secondary but can become primary following dental surgery. Teeth, particularly filled teeth, fit the classical definition of a focus as forming 'non-

absorbable material present in the connective tissue'.

Expert dental opinion is essential in order to deal with dental foci adequately, as in complicated cases dental surgery is often needed. The most likely teeth to act as a focus are root filled or devitalized teeth. BER techniques can establish which teeth are acting as a focus and thus help the dentist to locate those that need attention. In some cases complex homoeopathy alone can resolve many dental foci particularly where the problem is a chronic gingivitis or a similar condition.

Dental amalgam is a common source of trouble, and can often become toxic. Removal of dental amalgam and replacement with non-metallic fillings can produce enormously beneficial results in a wide variety of cases ranging from disseminated sclerosis to inflammation of the prostate gland. It cannot, however, be taken that removal of all dental amalgam in everybody is going to be uniformly beneficial. It is essential to make appropriate measurements using BER techniques to decide if the teeth are acting as a focus and if removal of dental amalgam would be beneficial. The number of patients in whom dental amalgam is a significant problem compared to the total numbers of people with dental amalgam fillings is very, very small indeed. It is therefore necessary to get the comments made here about the teeth in some sort of proportion. If the case is overstated then this simply detracts from the credibility of the original argument.

Dental foci can be important in many cases of facial pain, which are often grouped together under the unhelpful title of 'atypical facial pain'. Atypical facial pain basically means facial pain of unknown causation. BER techniques are able to make a correct diagnosis in a number of these cases, and the recommendation of appropriate dental work followed by long-term pain relief is always gratifying.

Salmonella Toxicity

Salmonella toxicity can occur after an infection with one of the salmonella bacteria such as Salmonella typhi, Salmonella paratyphi or Salmonella enteritidis. This gives the clinical picture of severe enteritis and often occurs in epidemics due to contaminated food. Salmonella toxicity can also come from ingesting Salmonella toxin present in processed food, most commonly tinned salmon, and BER techniques would lead one to believe that this is perhaps a commoner occurrence than many public health officials would care to admit.

The history is commonly of an initial gastroenteritis contracted whilst on holiday. In the United Kingdom this often occurs following holidays in Spain. The acute episode usually resolves spontaneously but may require appropriate antibiotic therapy. Following this the patient may well become chronically ill. The organs most likely to be damaged by Salmonella toxicity are the colon, liver, gall bladder, pancreas and heart.

Most people cope with Salmonella infection adequately; in others the toxins are released from the Salmonella organisms, enter the lymphatic system and overwhelm it with an excessive toxic load. As a result the toxins are deposited in the connective tissue. Here they remain locked away causing slow, insidious and persistent irritation at the sites where they are 'locked in'. This in turn can lead to chronic illness.

Complex homoeopathy offers an effective way of treating Salmonella toxicity by administering a nosode made from Salmonella to stimulate the body to excrete the Salmonella toxins from the cells in which they are locked. Also normal bacteria can be restored by giving appropriate live preparations of normal bacteria together with supportive therapy to whatever organs are stressed. In this case it is most likely to be the colon, liver and pancreas.

Streptococcal Toxicity

Infections due to streptococci are very common indeed. Usually occurring as tonsillitis, pharyngitis, tracheo-bronchitis, pneumonia, abscess or scarlet fever (rarer than some years previously). The acute infection is usually adequately dealt with by the administration of antibiotics of the penicillin group. In a few patients the toxin produced by the Streptococcal bacteria produces widespread damage to the immune system starting smouldering, insidious auto-immune damage to the body (this is a situation where the body seems to attack its own tissues).

The biggest group of diseases due to Streptococcal toxicity are the rheumatic diseases such as rheumatoid arthritis. Next comes rheumatic heart disease. In fact, any organ or tissue in the body may become involved in a chronic, low grade so-called auto-immune inflammatory process.

Conventional medicine has many reliable blood tests in order to detect Streptococcal toxicity. BER techniques are also useful and this is one of the few areas where both conventional and BER investigations often coincide.

In spite of the clear understanding of the diagnosis of Streptococcal toxicity by conventional medicine, conventional treatment still centres around giving steroids and/or immune suppressant drugs. In the patient with post-streptococcal rheumatoid arthritis pain is usually treated symptomatically using analgesics combined with anti-inflammatory drugs. In other words, even in a situation where the pathological progression is known, treatment is still not causally directed. Complex homoeopathy using nosodes made from Streptococci together with relevant appropriate therapy enables the cause to be treated directly.

Post-Viral States
Post-viral states are very common and usually occur following influenza, glandular fever and various other rarer conditions such as myalgic encephalomyelitis.

General and often debilitating fatigue is a common sequel to many viral infections, particularly the ones mentioned. The organs most commonly found to be stressed in these cases are the liver and pancreas. Complex homoeopathy, together with nutritional methods, is often an effective way of treating these conditions. Treatment centres around giving the patient a nosode of the original infecting virus together with complex homoeopathic therapy for the stressed organs. Often nutritional therapy in the form of vitamin and mineral replacements is also required in order to build up the patient's general resistance and to restore the body's often chronically depleted enzyme systems.

Conclusion
The conditions described in this chapter are of some importance as they are common underlying problems in many chronic diseases. A recognition of these underlying causes and their successful treatment is the key to long-lasting and fundamental improvement in many chronic illnesses which conventional medicine finds difficult to cope with, other than using a suppressive approach.

11. Self-Treatment Using Complex Homoeopathy

Much of this book has been about ideas, new technology and new concepts in medicine. This chapter is a simple patients' guide to the use of complex homoeopathy for a number of common ailments. The remedies are safe and over-dosage will do no harm although it is recommended that the stated dose should be adhered to.

General Principles
All remedies which work on the digestive organs such as the liver, gall bladder, pancreas, stomach and intestines should be taken about ten minutes before meals. They should be dropped onto the tongue or put in a glass of water and swallowed. Since complex homoeopathic remedies are relatively unpalatable their taste has to be disguised sometimes, especially for children. This be can done by placing them in orange juice or any other similar drink. As a general rule it is advisable to take liver remedies separate from other remedies. All the other before meal remedies can be mixed.

All remedies that are not for the liver, pancreas, colon, stomach, gall bladder or intestines, should be taken preferably 10 minutes after meals. It is advisable not to drink coffee or use toothpaste within half an hour of taking a complex remedy. This is not quite so important as in classical homoeopathy but is something which should be observed in order to ensure maximum efficiency of the medications. Allopathic medicaments which may be required (pain-killers etc.) may be taken at the same time as the complex homoeopathic remedies, but it is perferable to take these remedies without additional conventional drugs. This just isn't possible for some patients so a compromise must be reached.

Nosodes should only be given under properly trained supervision. They are usually rubbed into a soft area of the skin (such as around the navel) from where they are easily absorbed into the body. They are usually taken every other morning, but depending on the sensitivity of the patient this may have to be reduced to as little as once a week.

Dosage
Most complex homoeopathic preparations are available as drops — and this means that it is fairly easy to find the optimal dose by trial and error, in any particular situation. This is more difficult to do with tablets. The recommended dose in adults is 10 drops three times a day, before or after meals depending on which sort of remedy it is. In children below the age of fifteen the dose should be reduced to 5 drops and infants below two years to 2 drops, all three times a day. In this dosage system 1 tablet equals 5 drops, and so the correct dose of tablets for adults would be 2 three times a day, for children 1 tablet and lastly for infants ½ a tablet. The reason that the dosage frequency is three times a day is that complex homoeopathic remedies contain herbal medicaments and low potency homoeopathics, and as a consequence the preparation only acts for some five hours or so.

The recommended dose for nosodes is 5 drops, but considerable skill is required in order to get the dosage of nosode right and many factors have to be taken into consideration to determine this. This is why they are best taken under proper supervision.

Therapy for Specific Problems
The preparations referred to in this section are all made by Pascoe Pharmaceuticals of West Germany. (see Appendix). There are a number of other suppliers of complex homoeopathic preparations, the vast majority of whom are German Pharmaceutical Companies (see Appendix) and their products are all equally as good as the ones mentioned in this section. The reason for choosing the Pascoe Pharmacopoeia is that all their prescription books have now been translated into English and are therefore more accessible to readers of this book. The dosages given throughout this section refer to the adult dose.

When testing many patients using BER techniques it has been found that the most commonly stressed organs are the liver, pancreas and colon. In practice this means that in many diseases treatment using preparations acting on these organs is likely to be effective.

Preparations acting on the liver
Note that liver preparations tend to be poorly tolerated.

Lycopodium Similiaplexe	10 drops 3 times a day before meals.
Hepaticum tablets	1 tablet 3 times a day before meals. (Useful if constipation is present.)
Hepar Pasc tablets	1 tablet 3 times a day before meals. (Useful if the gall bladder is also involved.)
Cholesterinum Similaplexe	10 drops 3 times a day before meals. (Useful if the gall bladder is involved.)

Preparations acting on the pancreas

Pascopancreat drops	10 drops 3 times a day before meals. (This is the strongest pancreatic stimulant.)
Phaseolus Similiaplexe	10 drops 3 times a day before meals. (Useful for children.)
Carbo Vegetabilis Similiaplexe	10 drops 3 times a day before meals.

Preparations acting on the colon

Dysbiosan tablets	1 tablet 3 times a day before meals. (These tablets contain cascara as a mild laxative and some acidophilus bacteria. As this preparation also contains brewer's yeast it should not be used by individuals who are yeast sensitive.)
Markalakt powder	1 teaspoon dissolved in a glass of warm water 3 times a day before meals. (Useful for children. Contains Chamomile powder).

Specific Conditions

Acne Vulgaris
Acneiform Comedones are formed by the skin's sebaceous glands, this occurs in young adults and affects the face, chest and skin.

Causes: Acne appears to occur in patients who eat poor diets, have an essentially seborrhoeic skin, suffer from hormonal dysfunction, constipation, focal infection, and dysbiosis.

Types: Various stages of acne can be observed, from blackheads (comedones) to pustules and abscesses. These may be solitary or multiple.

Differential Diagnosis: Acneiform irritation caused by chemicals such as iodine, bromine and chlorine.

General Therapy: The metabolism should be regulated by draining out all the toxins and stabilizing the intestinal bacteria. Fresh air, plenty of sun, saunas and careful regular skin hygiene are all of value.

Diet: A lacto-vegetarian diet which involves raw food is helpful and this can be interspersed with fruit juice fasts. Pork, bacon, eggs and white sugar are all to be avoided.

Basic Therapy: Stropheupas-forte. 15 drops 3 times daily after meals.

Irritable Skin Conditions: Sulfur Similiaplexe: 2 tablets on the tongue daily; should an initial deterioration occur, reduce to 1 tablet once daily.

To accellerate resorption of hard skin abscesses in the early phases: Mercur. Sol. Similiaplexe: Allow 1 to 2 tablets to dissolve in the mouth 3 to 5 times daily.

To accelerate the maturation of abscesses where spots are not 'heading up': Hepar Sulf Similiaplexe: Allow 2 tablets to dissolve in the mouth hourly.

To help the liver excrete and deal with toxins: Legapas: ½ to 1 teaspoon in a ½ cup of warm water in the mornings. *Hepaticum-Pascoe:* 3 tablets to be swallowed whole morning and afternoon in warm water.

To overcome constipation and purge the intestines: Pascolletten: 1 to 2 tablets twice daily.

To re-establish bacterial equilibrium in the intestines: Markalakt:

1 teaspoon in 1 cup of warm water in the morning taken on an empty stomach. *Dysbiosan:* 1 to 2 tablets, 2 to 3 times a day to be taken ½ hour before meals. (*Dysbiosan* contains normal intestinal bacteria.) For further normalization of bowel bacteria see Chapter 9. Depending on the individual situation each person with acne should be able to decide which combination of remedies is most appropriate for their particular case.

Angina Pectoria
This usually presents itself as an attack of severe chest pain occurring on the left side radiating down towards the abdomen, up into the left side of the neck or down the left arm. Associated symptoms of collapse and severe anxiety may be present.

Organic Causes:

1   Coronary artery disease.
2   Cardiac insufficiency.

Functional Causes:

1   Coronary artery spasm following physical exertion, nicotine abuse, severe exposure to hydrocarbon chemicals in sensitive individuals, and severe anxiety.
2   High blood-pressure.
3   Kidney disease.
4   Enterocardiac symptom complex (Roemheld's syndrome)*.

Differential Diagnosis: Heart attack, in such instances there will be no improvement with taking *Glycryl trinitrate* sublingually (the most common method of providing immediate relief for angina).

General Therapy: Regular intestinal evacuation, breathing exercises (particularly diaphragmatic breathing which results in increased arterial blood oxygen level).

Physical Therapy: Regular light exercise.

*Roemheld's syndrome: A syndrome due to excess gas production in the abdomen described by Dr Roemheld. The excess gas splints and raises the diaphragm which in turn alters the axis of the heart and thereby affects its function.

Diet: Should be lacto-vegetarian with plenty of raw food and lots of fruit.

Acute angina: Glycryl trinitrate sublingually — 1 to 2 tablets as necessary.

Treatment for chronic angina:

Basic Therapy: Pectapas drops: 10 to 20 drops 2 to 3 times daily after meals.

To improve coronary blood supply: Stropheupas-forte. 20 drops in a tablespoon of water 1 to 3 times daily after meals. *Cactus Grandiflorus Similiaplexe:* 10 to 15 drops 3 times daily after meals.

In the initial stages of cardiac insufficiency (cardiac failure): *Viscorapas:* 1 to 3 tablets 3 times daily after meals.

For Percutaneous Therapy: Percutaneous *Pectapas* ointment: 1 to 2 cm ointment rubbed over the region of the heart morning and evening.

Preventive treatment in cases of anxiety: Seda-pasc: 2 tablets 3 times daily after meals.

For pain radiating into the left arm and left side of the neck: Spigelia Similiaplexe: 10 to 15 drops daily after meals.

Chest pain associated with high blood pressure: Arnica Montana Similiaplexe: 15 drops in water at 10am, 4pm and 8pm in conjunction with *Spartium Similiaplexe:* 10 to 40 drops 1 to 3 times daily after meals.

As a daytime sedative if there is a tendency for Roemheld's symptom complex (this would invariably require expert attention to diagnosis as to whether this is present or not): *Pasconal-forte:* 10 to 20 drops 1 to 6 times daily. (Collections of gas in the abdomen can trigger off an acute angina attack.) *Pascopankreat* drops or tablets: 1 to 2 tablets, yellow before and red during and after meals, swallowed whole with water, or 10 to 30 drops three times daily 10 to 15 minutes before meals.

Arthritis

Arthritis means acute or chronic inflammation of the joints.

1   Acute arthritis — solitary, inflammatory or infective.
2   Acute polyarthritis — rheumatoid arthritis, acute rheumatism.
3   Chronic arthritis — usually affects a single joint such as a knee or a hip.
4   Chronic polyarthritis — 'wear and tear' arthritis affecting a number of joints.
5   Gout — associated with a high level of uric acid in the blood.
6   Arthrosis deformans — a combination of degenerative and proliferative processes in the cartilage and bone resulting in gross physical deformity of the joint involved.

Differential Diagnosis: A tubercular or fungal infection of the joint. Psoriatic arthritis.

General Therapy: Flush the toxins out through the skin. Cantharide plasters on the affected joints can be useful as can diaphoretic therapy to help the patient to sweat toxins out through the skin. Taking a bath (as hot as can be tolerated) with some Epsom Salts added can help in this regard. Toxins can also be removed from the body by purging. Acupuncture is probably the most effective local treatment.

1. Acute arthritis:

For internal therapy of acute inflammation and resorption of fluid from a joint: Ranunculus Similiaplexe — 10 to 15 drops hourly in conjunction with *Rheuma-pasc* — ½ to 1 teaspoonful 3 times daily. *Ledum Similiaplexe* 10 drops hourly.

As a diuretic to drain the toxins from the body: Juniperus Similiaplexe 10 drops 3 times daily taken in a small glass of water. *Berberis-tonic* 1 teaspoonful 3 times a day.

2. Acute polyarthritis:

As well as the therapy suggested above, the following are useful:

For specific and anti-toxic therapy: nosodes may well have to be used. In this situation an appropriately qualified practitioner should be contacted.

To increase the body's resistance to infection in feverish conditions: Bryonia-forte Similiaplexe: 10 to 15 drops in a tablespoonful of water, hourly, together with *Pascotox* (tablets or drops): 1 dose of 60 drops, or 10 tablets on the tongue with a subsequent hourly dose of 20 drops or 2 tablets.

In cases of rheumatic neuralgia: Aconitum Similiaplexe: 10 to 20 drops every hour, *Dioscorea Similiaplexe:* 10 drops 3 to 6 times daily.

For treatment of acute bouts of infection: Rhus Toxicodendron Similiaplexe: 10 to 20 drops 3 times daily.

3. Chronic arthritis and
4. Chronic polyarthritis:

Basic diuretic therapy for drainage of toxins: Berberis Similiaplexe 20 drops 3 times daily in a small glass of water. *Rheumapasc* tablets may also be used.

For specific anti-toxic therapy: A nosode complex may have to be used for this and an appropriately qualified practitioner should be contacted.

For the treatment of Gout: Ledum Similiaplexe: 10 to 20 drops 3 times daily.

For joint swelling: Colchicum Similiaplexe: 10 to 20 drops 3 times daily.

Follow up treatment of chronic arthritis in order to correct the acid base balance in the tissues: Acidum Oxalicum Similiaplexe: 10 to 15 drops 1 to 3 times daily.

5. Gout:
Basic diuretic therapy to drain toxins: Berberis Similiaplexe: 20 drops 3 times daily in a small glass of water. Also *Berberis* tonic.

Specific treatment in cases of raised blood uric acid (gout): Acidum Oxalicum Similiaplexe: 10 to 15 drops 1 to 3 times daily.

Specific therapy for a gouty joint: Ledum Similiaplexe: 15 drops 3 times daily alternating with *Colchicum Similiaplexe:* 10 to 15 drops 3 times daily.

6. Arthrosis deformans:
Basic Therapy: Rheumapasc: ½ to 1 tablespoonful 3 times daily.

Asthma
1. Bronchial Asthma: In bronchial asthma there is difficulty in expiration due to contraction of the smooth muscles in the walls of the bronchi (breathing tubes) together with associated secretion of sticky mucus into the bronchial tree.

Causes: Allergic reactions to inhaled substances, chemicals and ingested foods. Associated with colonic dysfunction (dysbacteria and dysbiosis) pyschological problems, irritability of the autonomic nervous system consequent on chronic lung disease such as severe chest infection. Bronchial asthma is particularly associated with focal infections of the sinuses and appendix.

Differential Diagnosis: Cardiac asthma (left ventricular failure) and uraemia (a conditions where the kidneys are failing and there are high circulating levels of blood urea which is normally excreted in the urine).

General Therapy:

1 Breathing Exercises, autogenic training. (See Chapter 6).
2 Drain out toxins by promoting a diuresis through the kidneys (i.e. increasing urine flow).
3 Acupuncture.
4 Treatment of an underlying dysbacteria or dysbiosis if it is present.
5 Treatment of relevant foci which may involve appendicectomy if an underlying focus is the appendix and does not respond to conservative therapy.

Diet: Diet should be rich in lactates and should be free from any obvious allergens. The asthmatic patient may well have to be tested for food and airborne sensitivities (see *Clinical Ecology* by George T. Lewith and Julian Kenyon, published by Thorsons, 1985).

Therapy in Bronchial Asthma: Asthmapas drops: 10 to 15 drops 3 times daily. In an acute attack 20 to 40 drops taken hourly. *Yerba Santa Similiaplexe:* 10 to 15 drops 1 to 3 times daily.

2. Asthma associated with an irritating nocturnal cough:
Hyoscyamus Similiaplexe: 15 to 20 drops twice before sleeping.

As a percutaneous expectorant: Palatol: Rub 10 to 20 drops into the chest or the back, wait until the *Palatol* has been absorbed and the skin appears dry again.

To support the heart and circulation: Viscorapas: 2 tablets with some water 3 times daily.

To promote expectoration of sticky mucus: Cetraria Islandica Similiaplexe: 10 to 15 drops 1 to 3 times daily.

3. Cardiac Asthma:
In attacks of cardiac asthma the shortage of breath which nearly always occurs in the early hours of the morning is associated with failure of the left side of the heart and the consequent lung congestion due to blood damming up in the lung circulation.

The treatment of cardiac failure: Viscorapas: 2 tablets taken with some water 3 times daily, *Cardiacum II:* 10 drops 3 times daily. In all cases of cardiac asthma proper medical opinion should be sought as the measures recommended may not be powerful enough to cope with severe cardiac asthma.

Bed-wetting (Enuresis):
In most patients who complain of persistent enuresis a congenital or acquired weakness of the bladder is present. It is important to consider other causes however, such as kidney stones, spina bifida occulta, chronic constipation, generalized endocrine disturbances (often initiated by geopathic stress) and epilepsy.

General Therapy: Exclude drinks from 5 pm onwards. Use dry foods for the evening meal. The child should be woken 2 or 3 times during the night and encouraged to pass water. Other treatments which can be of value include food allergy testing, acupuncture and psychotherapy.

Basic Therapy for Enuresis: Clematis Similiaplexe: 10 to 15 drops in a teaspoonful of water 2 to 3 times daily. For bladder weakness: *Solidago Similiaplexe:* 10 to 15 drops in a small glass of water 3 times daily.

In cases where there is kidney stress following acute or chronic Nephritis (inflammation of the kidney): *Juniperus Similiaplexe:* 10 to 15 drops in water 3 times daily. *Pascorenal:* 3 to 5 drops in water 2 times daily increasing by 1 drop per day up to 15 to 20 drops 3 times daily.

For Enuresis associated with intestinal worm infestation: Abrotanum Similiaplexe: 2 to 12 drops 1 to 2 times daily according to the age of the child (increase by one drop for every year).

Catarrh
In cases of inflammation of the upper respiratory tract:

As a preventive: Gripps (drops): children 20 to 40 drops, adults 40 to 80 drops in a small glass of water from which a sip should be taken every 15 to 30 minutes.

In order to clear the respiratory passages: Eupatorium Similiaplexe: 10 drops every ½ to 1 hour alternating with *Bryonia Forte Similiaplexe:* 15 drops in a tablespoonful of water every half hour.

For symptomatic treatment of a cough: Tussiflorin drops: 15 to 20 drops in a tablespoonful of water 3 to 4 times a day.

To increase the body's powers of resistance: Pascotox tablets and drops: 1 dose of 60 drops or 10 tablets on the tongue with subsequent hourly doses of 20 drops or 2 tablets.

As a percutaneous expectorant: Palatol: rub 15 to 20 drops into the chest and back, wait until the *Palatol* is absorbed and the skin appears to be dry again. *Palatol* is also available as an ointment in which case 1 to 2 cms of cream should be rubbed in.

Cholecystitis
Cause: Acute inflammation of the bile ducts and gall bladder following an ascending infection, a blood borne infection or gall stones and pancreatitis.

Symptoms: Temperature associated with rigors. The gall bladder is often enlarged and painful to touch if the upper right part of the abdomen just below the ribs is palpitated. There are often severe colicky pains radiating from the right upper part of the abdomen into the back and under the right shoulder-blade which are associated with nausea, sometimes jaundice, and indigestion particularly aggravated by fatty foods.

Differential Diagnosis: Appendicitis, pleurisy, renal colic, other acute and chronic diseases of the liver and gastric and duodenal ulcers.

General Therapy: Fasting, regular defaecation and avoidance of foods to which the patient may be sensitive. (This has to be determined by prior testing.) Hot, damp compresses can be of value placed over the sight of the pain and also over the equivalent place on the right-hand side of the back.

Diet: A light diet rich in carbohydrates and low in fats and proteins is recommended. Animal fats should be avoided as should alcohol, coffee, tea and cigarette smoking. Fruit, vegetable juices, buttermilk, curdled milk and small quantities of chilled sunflower oil are recommended.

To combat infection and increase the body's powers of resistance: Bryonia Similiaplexe: 10 to 15 drops in a tablespoonful of water every ½ to 1 hour, if appropriate, alternating with *Pascotox* (tablets and drops): 1 dose of 60 drops or 10 tablets on the tongue with subsequent hourly doses of 20 drops or 2 tablets.

To reduce the spasm in the bile ducts in cases of acute biliary colic: Carduus Marianus Similiaplexe: 8 to 10 drops at 1 to 15 minute intervals alternating with *Colocynthis Similiaplexe:* 2 tablets on the tongue every 5 to 15 minutes.

When the gall bladder ceases to function correctly: *Cholesterinum Similiaplexe:* 10 to 15 drops 3 times daily.

To normalize bile secretion: Hepaticum Pascoe: 2 to 4 tablets twice daily.

To tonify and protect the liver from damage: Hepar Pasc: 2 tablets 1 to 3 times daily.

Climacteric (menopausal problems)
Basic Therapy: Vicordin-elixir: 1 teaspoonful 3 times daily.
Oophorinum complex drops: 10 drops 1 to 3 times daily.

For hot flushes: Sanguinaria Similiaplexe: 10 drops 1 to 3 times daily.

For dizziness: Glonoinum Similiaplexe: 10 to 15 drops 3 times daily.

For headaches and ringing in the ears associated with the menopause: Cimicifuga Similiaplexe: 10 to 15 drops 1 to 3 times daily.

As a tonic: Hocura-feminina: 1 tablespoonful 3 times daily.

Constipation
The cause of constipation must be defined and treated. A high-fibre diet is the mainstay of therapy. Hydrotherapy, breathing exercises and enemas can also be of value.

For the treatment of constipation associated with portal venous congestion (high pressure in the liver circulation): *Legapas:* ½ to 1 teaspoonful in half a cup of warm water.

For the treatment of habitual constipation: Pascoletten: 2 to 3 tablets in the evening.

Cystitis
This is acute or chronic inflammation of the bladder and the ureter. In men it is most commonly caused by Streptococcal infection and in women by E. coli (these are two common sorts of bacteria).

Symptoms: Painful, burning frequent urination. If the upper part of the kidney tract is infected then there may be rigors, sweating, vomiting and shooting pains in the area of the loins. There may be some blood and pus in the urine.

Differential Diagnosis: Appendicitis, cholecystitis, pneumonia, tuberculosis affecting the urinary tract, kidney or bladder stones or disease of the kidneys.

General Therapy: Bed rest for the first few days with local application of warmth over the loins. Fluid intake should be encouraged including the liberal use of herb teas. Antibiotic therapy is often indicated in the chronic situation.

Diet: Fruit juices and a lacto-vegetarian diet are advisable. Alcohol and nicotine are forbidden.

Basic Therapy for Cystitis: Solidago Similiaplexe: 10 to 15 drops in a small glass of water 3 to 6 times daily alternating with *Cantharis Similiaplexe* 8 to 10 drops 3 to 6 times daily.

Basic Therapy in chronic Cystitis: Clematis Similiaplexe: 10 to 15 drops in a teaspoonful of water 3 times daily.

If a temperature and rigors are present: Bryonia Forte Similiaplexe: 10 to 20 drops in a tablespoonful of water every 1 to 2 hours.

To increase the body's power of resistance: Pascotox tablets or drops: initial dose of 60 drops or 10 tablets on the tongue with subsequent hourly doses of 20 drops or 2 tablets.

If there is an accompanying infection of the kidney: Juniperus Similiaplexe: 10 to 15 drops in a teaspoonful of water 3 times daily. *Pascorenal:* 20 to 30 drops in hot water 3 times daily.

In cases where there is an accompanying prostatitis (inflammation of the prostate gland): *Populus Similiaplexe:* 10 to 15 drops 3 times daily, *Pascosabal:* 20 drops in hot water 3 times daily.

Dysmenorrhoea (painful periods)
Causes:

1 Organic causes such as salipingitis (inflammation of the uterus and tubes), fibroids, polyps, tumours in the female genital tract, prolapse, local scarring and in some cases a retroverted (backwards lying) uterus.
2 Functional conditions such as endocrine disturbances and emotional problems.

General Therapy:

1 Drain the toxins via the kidneys and intestines.
2 Hot sitz baths (baths where the patient sits with the pelvis in a

tub of very hot water) with the addition of Epsom salts or similar to promote increased blood flow to the pelvis and also local sweating.

3   Acupuncture: The spleen meridian, in particular spleen 6, is an effective point.

4   Testing food sensitivities can be useful in some cases of dysmenorrhoea.

5   Supplementation with zinc and vitamin B_6 can be effective.

Basic treatment of dysmenorrhoea: Pulsatilla Similiaplexe: 10 to 15 drops 1 to 3 times daily in conjunction with *Hocura-feminina:* 1 tablespoonful 3 times daily.

In cases of congested pelvic circulation associated with constipation: Petroselinum Similiaplexe: 2 to 3 tablets daily starting about 3 to 5 days before the period is expected.

Dyspepsia
The disturbance of digestion either in the stomach or the upper part of the small intestine. Frequently there is a dysfermentia (abnormal bacterial fermentation caused by abnormal intestinal bacteria).

Symptoms: Anorexia, flatulence, heartburn and distended upper abdomen. Dyspepsia may be a symptom of many diseases and consequently an accurate diagnosis must be made.

General Therapy: A diet which clears residual toxicity out of the system consisting of freshly roasted, freshly ground and filtered real coffee without milk or sugar. Avoid nicotine and alcohol.

Basic Therapy: Amara drops: 25 drops in the morning on an empty stomach and a cup of real coffee as recommended above or 15 to 20 drops 3 times daily, quarter of an hour before meals. (Some patients are sensitive to coffee and will not be able to follow the instructions for drinking real coffee).

To normalize pancreatic function and the treatment of anorexia: Pascopankreat drops and tablets: 1 to 2 tablets at midday and in the evening, yellow before and red during and after the meals, to be swallowed whole with some liquid. Alternatively, take 10 to 30 drops in a small glass of water 3 times daily 10 to 15 minutes before meals.

To treat abdominal distention and heartburn: Dysbiosan: 1 to 2 tablets 2 to 3 times daily to be taken half an hour before meals. *Pascomag* (powder): 1 teaspoonful of powder 3 times daily with water before meals.

Eczema
This is an irritant and inflammatory condition of the skin. Eczematous areas usually heal without scar formation.

1   Toxic Eczema: this is produced by direct effect of a strong irritant on the skin, such as a chemical.
2   Allergic Eczema:
    (a) Eczema resulting from the absorption of intestinal toxins. This is often associated with a dysbiosis.
    (b) Eczema caused by external agents:
        (i) Contact eczema or contact dermatitis following contact with allergens such as detergents, cosmetics, allergenic foods and various metals such as nickel.
        (ii) Contact with microbial parasitic products such as bacteria, fungi and lice.
3   Seborrhoeic Eczema: eczema complicated by irritant products produced by skin metabolism such as sweat, skin oils, etc.

Eczema is an allergic disease which can only be treated successfully if the cause if defined. It is very important in all cases of eczema to test for food sensitivities and also for house dust and dust mite sensitivity.

The most important therapy for contact eczema is to discover and exclude the allergic substance. If the skin is affected by fungi and bacteria then the external application of appropriate allopathic therapeutic creams is required.

For general therapy: (as Eczema is largely an allergic complaint the treatment here is that of allergy): *Pascallerg* tablets: Acute: allow 2 tablets to dissolve in the mouth every 1 to 2 hours, Chronic: allow 2 tablets to dissolve in the mouth 3 times daily. Nosode therapy is often important in all allergies and appropriate help should be sought in order to select the correct nosode complexes required.

To detoxify and improve liver metabolism: Quassia Similiaplexe: 10 to 15 drops in a teaspoonful of water 3 times daily in conjunction with *Legapas:* in cases of constipation following insufficient gall bladder activity ¼ to ½ teaspoonful in ½ cup of warm water. *Hepar-pasc:* (In cases of liver damage) 1 to 2 tablets twice daily with some water.

Treatment of accompanying Dyspepsia and Dysfermentia: Amara drops: 15 drops 3 times daily in water, *Pascopankreat* tablets or drops: 1 to 2 yellow tablets before evening and midday meals and 1 to 2 red ones during and after meals, swallowed whole with some water: or 10 to 30 drops in quarter of a glass of warm water 3 times daily 10 to 15 minutes before meals.

For the treatment of accompanying dysbacteria: Ozovit: 1 teaspoonful twice daily with warm water between meals. *Markalakt:* 1 teaspoonful in a cup of hot water in the morning on an empty stomach. *Dysbiosan:* 1 to 2 tablets 2 to 3 times a day to be taken half an hour before meals.

Gastroenteritis
Causes: Contaminated food, laxative abuse, over-indulgence in alcohol, tobacco, sweet or very fatty foods, chemical and other intoxications.

Symptoms: Gastroenteritis is non-specific inflammation of the lining membranes of the stomach and intestinal canal, usually causing diarrhoea and vomiting. It is the body's way of clearing out toxic products.

Differential Diagnosis: Dysentry, paratyphus, cholera.

General Therapy: Short periods of purging. One to two days of fasting on herb teas and the use of charcoal can help. Diet in general should be light, eating fresh fruit such as grated apples. Keep the abdomen warm and dry; dry compresses may help. Bed rest is advisable. Acupuncture can be helpful.

Detoxification treatment in order to clear out the intestines: Pascoletten: 2 to 3 tablets as a single dose. To treat acute intestinal upsets: *China Similiaplexe:* 10 drops in water taken hourly.

If Gastroenteritis is accompanied by temperature: *Nux Vomica Similiaplexe:* 10 to 15 drops 3 to 6 times daily alternating with *Bryonia Forte Similiaplexe:* 10 to 15 drops in a tablespoon of water 3 to 6 times daily.

In cases of associated pancreatic dysfunction and flatulence: *Pascopankreat* tablets and drops: At midday and the evenings 1 to 2 tablets, yellow before and red during and after meals, swallowed whole with some water: or 10 to 30 drops 3 times daily in quarter of a glass of warm water 10 to 15 minutes before meals.

Basic Therapy during a period of fast: Markalakt: 1 teaspoonful in a cup of warm water 3 times daily. *Muscopas* tablets: 4 to 8 tablets with water 3 times daily. *Dysbiosan:* 1 to 2 tablets 2 to 3 times daily to be taken half an hour before meals.

Haemorrhoids
Causes: Constitutional weakness of blood vessels and congestion in the portal (liver) circulation. Haemorrhoids are associated with constipation, liver disease, a sedentary lifestyle, pregnancy and cardiac failure.

Symptoms: Anal irritation, anal pain, particularly on defaecation and when sitting on a cold surface. Bleeding is a major complication.

Differential Diagnosis: The possibility of a rectal cancer should be excluded by appropriate medical examination.

General Therapy: Regular bowel movement and clearing the portal circulation. Anal hygiene is also important.

Local Therapy: Anisan Haemorrhoidal Suppositories: 1 suppository twice daily. *Anisan* Haemorrhoidal ointment.

To treat abnormal portal circulation: Pascovenol drops: 20 drops 3 times daily before meals.

To normalize liver metabolism and clear out the intestines: Legapas: ½ to 1 teaspoonful in half a glass of warm water in the morning, *Lycopodium Similiaplexe:* 10 drops 1 to 3 times daily before meals. *Hepaticum-Pascoe:* 2 to 3 tablets with water in the morning and afternoon, *Pascoletten:* 1 to 3 tablets in the evening.

Hay fever
This is an allergic reaction due to sensitivity to pollens from flowers, grasses, weeds and trees. It usually occurs between May and August.

See under the section for eczema (allergy). Homoeopathic potencies of the specific pollens can also be useful. These should be given under the direction of a qualified homoeopath.

Headaches

Headache is a frequent complaint and it is essential to establish a proper diagnosis by consulting a qualified doctor.

For Symptomatic Therapy: Pascodolor: 1 to 2 powders in water. *Iris Similiaplexe:* 10 to 20 drops hourly 3 times daily alternating with *Gelsemium Similiaplexe:* 10 drops 3 times daily.

To rub over the affected area: Palatol: Rub 5 to 10 drops.

Laryngitis

Differential Diagnosis: laryngeal infection, laryngeal nodes, laryngeal cancer (very rare).

General Therapy: No smoking and the use of soothing inhalations. Promote the excretion of toxins from the kidney. Hot compresses on the neck will stimulate sweating and clear the toxins through the skin.

For acute Laryngitis: Arum Similiaplexe: 10 drops 3 times daily alternating with *Drosera Similiaplexe:* 10 to 30 drops on a sugar lump 3 times daily.

For inhalation therapy: Palatol: 5 to 10 drops in 1 chamomile steam bath (*Markalakt* powder contains chamomile and can be used to add to a steam bath).

Drainage of the toxins from the kidneys: Pascorenol: 50 to 100 drops in a tablespoonful of water 3 times daily.

For local therapy: Palatol ointment: rub into the area of the neck several times daily.

Menorrhagia (heavy periods)

If this condition is persistent, then proper medical opinion should be sought. Among the possible causes are: uterine prolapse, ovarian tumours, polyps, genital infections and uterine malignancy.

Cases of heavy regular bleeding with no serious underlying cause: Millefolium Similiaplexe: initially 30 to 40 drops in a teaspoonful of water: further hourly doses 10 to 20 drops, alternating with *Asperula Similiaplexe:* 10 to 20 drops every hour.

Migraine

Migraine headaches usually involve severe one-sided headaches associated with visual and occasional auditory disturbances, nausea and vomiting, dizziness and in several cases tinglings in various parts of the body. The possibility of a tumour in the head must be excluded although this is extremely rare.

Migraine in women: Often caused by pelvic, liver and gall bladder, intestinal and kidney dysfunction.

Migraine in men: Predominantly caused by dysfunction in the gastro-intestinal tract, the prostate and the kidneys.

Some cases of migraine are due to cervical spine arthritis in which case physical therapy such as acupuncture or manipulation is essential. In some patients migraine may be due to food sensitivity and therefore food testing is mandatory in all cases of migraine. (See *Clinical Ecology* by George Lewith and Julian Kenyon, published by Thorsons, 1985.)

Pains in the forehead associated with genital infection: Iris Similiaplexe alternating with *Apis Similiaplexe:* 10 drops 1 to 3 times daily.

Headaches associated with menstrual disturbances: Iris Similiaplexe alternating with *Cimicifuga Similiaplexe:* 10 drops 1 to 3 times daily.

Headaches associated with vaginal or uterine products: Iris Similiaplexe alternating with *Sepia Similiaplexe:* 10 drops 1 to 3 times daily.

Headaches occurring predominantly on the right: Carduus Marianus Similiaplexe, alternating with *Quassia Similiaplexe:* 10 drops 1 to 3 times daily.

Headaches occurring predominantly on the left: Iris Similiaplexe alternating with *China Similiaplexe:* 10 drops 1 to 3 times daily.

Headaches occurring in anxious individuals or in association with gastroenteritis: Iris Similiaplexe alternating with *Nux Vomica Similiaplexe* alternating with *Artemesia Similiaplexe:* 10 drops 1 to 2 times daily.

Headaches occurring in association with kidney dysfunction: Iris Similiaplexe alternating with *Juniperus Similiaplexe:* 10 drops 1 to 3 times daily.

Headaches occurring in association with high blood-pressure: Iris Similiaplexe alternating with *Arnica Similiaplexe* alternating with *Rutin Similiaplexe:* 10 drops 1 to 3 times daily. In cases of high blood-pressure a qualified medical opinion is essential.

Headaches occurring in association with hypotension (low blood-pressure): *Iris Similiaplexe* alternating with *Ambra Similiaplexe* alternating with *Glonoinum Similiaplexe:* 10 drops 1 to 3 times daily.

Headaches associated with neuralgic pains in the head and neck: Iris Similiaplexe alternating with *Aconitum Similiaplexe:* 10 drops 1 to 3 times daily.

Prostate Problems
The enlarged prostate:
Symptoms: Difficulty in passing water, poor stream and frequency.

Differential Diagnosis: Prostatitis (inflammation of the prostate gland), prostatic tuberculosis, prostatic carcinoma.

General Therapy: Use a lacto-vegetarian diet low in salt and spices. Regular bowel movements are important. Avoid cold drinks, alcohol and coffee. Hormonal therapy is of value as is surgery, if the case is advanced. It is important to exclude cancer of the prostate and therefore a qualified medical opinion is essential.

Basic Therapy: Pascosabal: 20 drops 3 times daily alternating with *Populus Similiaplexe* 10 drops 3 times daily. Rubbing *Lymphdiaral* ointment on to the prostate gland by inserting a finger into the lower end of the rectum, twice daily, is very useful.

To reduce enlargement of the prostate gland: Thuja Similiaplexe:

12. Response to Treatment Using Complex Homoeopathy

As complex homoeopathy is fundamentally a stimulatory therapeutic approach initial worsening in the patient's condition can sometimes occur. Usually this is short lived, lasting only a few days. If the worsening persists for more than a few days then the medication should be stopped, as the cause is likely to be intolerance to one or a number of the medicines.

As a rule, if therapy is successful there is a slow and continued improvement with perhaps a few ups and downs, particularly if the problem is an intermittent one like migraine or dysmenorrhoea. As a general rule any illness which has lasted more than a few years will take six to nine months to get better.

Response to Nosodes
These are homoeopathic dilutions of toxins and stimulate the cells to discharge the appropriate toxins into the extracellular fluid which surrounds the cells. Occasionally this discharge of toxins can produce an alarming response, which is why nosodes ought to be used only under the supervision of a properly trained practitioner. If the patient is very debilitated, such as in terminal cancer or is elderly and frail, then nosodes should not generally be used as the patient will be too weak to cope with an onrush of toxins released into the extracellular fluid, and in some cases the use of nosodes can lead to long lasting worsening.

Complex homoeopathy relies on washing the toxins released in this way out through the skin, urinary tract and colon. As a consequence it is not unusual for the urine to change colour, the bowels to become loose, or for the odour of the sweat to be unpleasant as the toxins are released. In some cases of sinusitis the sinuses may start to stream or when treating inflammation of the external ear (Otitis externa) the ear may start to discharge. All of these changes are good signs, as an initial worsening, as it shows that the body is doing something to expel toxins. The last thing to do is to suppress these reactions by taking anti-diarrhoea tablets or suppressing the flow of mucus from the sinuses. If the response is too much then simply reduce the dosage of the medicines.

What happens when there is no response to treatment?
The most disappointing result of all is when nothing happens. This either means that the therapy is wrong or there is a blocked treatment. Blocks to treatment are usually due to one of the following factors:

1   An underlying pyschological problem
2   Geopathic stress (Chapter 10)
3   A focus, such as a tooth or chronic appendicitis
    (see Chapter 5)
4   A very debilitated patient

In order for the patient to respond then the underlying problem needs to be recognized and tackled in an appropriate manner.

What about concurrent conventional treatment?
Usually people who come along with a chronic problem are already on conventional drugs. These should be continued, and in some cases it is dangerous to discontinue them suddenly, especially if a patient is on steroids, but the dose should gradually be reduced as the complex homoeopathy starts to work. Unfortunately steroids will depress the response to homoeopathy and it compromises the body's regulatory ability. Generally speaking it isn't possible to stop steroids suddenly, as there can be severe adrenal suppression as a result. Steroids therefore have to be reduced slowly and under medical supervision. Therapy in these patients will be much more drawn out than those who are not taking these drugs.

What if the patient continues to get worse?
If worsening persists for more than three to four days without any obvious cause other than the medication, then the first thing to do is to stop the nosode. If this does not improve things then stop the drops before meals and lastly the drops after meals. One or a number of these measures should stop any continued worsening.

The phenomenon of 'playback'
Some patients, whilst taking complex homoeopathy (or classical homoeopathy) replay their previous illnesses in abbrieviated form. It is important to recognize this when it does happen as it is invariably a good sign, so the patient must be encouraged to go through with it.

When should therapy be stopped?
As BER techniques always show some abnormality, no matter how healthy the patient is, then the decision when to stop treatment must be a clinical one. The wisest approach is to stop medications in stages, dropping the nosode first if one has been used, when all the clinical symptoms have disappeared or when as much improvement as possible has been achieved.

What about preventive medicine?
BER techniques can pick out pre-clinical illness, and the awkward question arises as to whether these methods can be used in preventive medicine. Clearly they can, but my own approach is mildly to discourage this practice until the methods and therapies are better proven or better developed (or both), otherwise there is a danger that this new approach to medicine will be killed stone dead before it has time to establish itself because of accusations of charlatanism.

Conclusion
Complex homoeopathic therapy produces an initial worsening in a small proportion of patients. The most worrying response is no change at all, and a reason must be sought for this. Treatment with complex homoeopathy is rather like peeling an onion; at each consultation another layer is peeled away revealing a slightly different clinical situation underneath. Therapy should be continuously modified to accommodate this changing state of the patient. How many layers of the onion to peel is a matter for clinical judgement.

14. Cancer Treatment

Cancer is regarded as the most serious of all diseases, and many people believe that it is synonymous with death. There is increasing dissatisfaction with conventional approaches to cancer, and it is not unusual to come across patients who have turned down all orthodox approaches in favour of the so called 'gentle' approach, characterized by the intensive use of a number of natural therapies. This would have been unheard of ten years ago. Conventional cancer treatment is drastic, negative and further injures the body. Not surprisingly, it is justifiably receiving much criticism, as it still shows a fragmented, uncoordinated approach to this poorly understood problem. Conventional treatment concentrates only on the tumour, as if it didn't exist within a patient. The psychological aspects of cancer, now fairly well accepted, are usually given lip service at best with no fundamental approach on this front. The patient, however, is just as much to blame as he tends to look at his tumour as something separate from himself which merely needs to be chopped off, and rarely considers the broader context of the illness. The alternative approaches to cancer, if nothing else, are forcing a broader view of cancer on patient and doctor alike. This change of approach is long overdue and has been vigorously resisted by conventional cancer doctors.

Diagnosis
Current diagnostic techniques in malignancy largely rely on looking for a 'lump' in the body. The level of confidence in these methods is well illustrated by a comment in *New Scientist*[1] concerning a statement made in April 1984 by the US National Cancer Institute (N.C.I.) which said that it had announced to the US Senate that, by the year 2000, it could and would halve the number of Americans who die of cancer. *New Scientist* commented that this aim would

be very difficult to achieve, saying that: 'All these claims are clearly admirable. But do the numbers make sense? The hopes for attacking micrometases (small secondary tumours) for instance, demand a great deal of optimism. We have no real way of knowing if the future holds better methods of detection or treatment of these cells. The prediction of a 30% reduction in mortality from the two proposed measures seems to be based on little more than faith in the brilliance and innovation of cancer researchers'. Clearly, therefore, the scientific community has little faith in the NCI's aim. This lack of faith is clearly reflected in the public's attitude to conventional cancer treatment. From all points of view a new approach is called for.

As far as diagnosis is concerned, continuing to concentrate on looking for physical damage in the body, no matter how small, is unlikely to produce a major advance in early diagnosis. BER techniques clearly indicate that looking for energetic change is a real possibility, the implication being that any cancer first starts as an energetic change in the body. As yet the findings of BER medicine in this area have not been tested for accuracy in diagnosis. Clearly this needs to be looked at as a matter of urgency, as without this it is difficult to know how much faith to put into BER findings which give a diagnosis of cancer. My own feeling is that the present technology available in BER medicine needs to be developed to much higher levels of sensitivity to offer any real hope of measuring objectively the subtle electrical changes indicated before and of course when a tumour exists in the body. Unfortunately, the current mechanistic reductionist 'mind-set' is set against any fundamental discoveries being made in this area, if only for the reason that adequate funding will be denied to these approaches. These ideas will be discussed more fully in the last chapter.

Causes of Cancer

With cancer, more than with any other illness, the traditional biomedical practice of associating a physical disease with a specific physical cause is inappropriate. But since most researchers still operate within the current biomedical framework, they find the phenomenon of cancer extremely bewildering. As a result cancer management today is in a state of confusion.

However, changes are gradually occurring in the way we perceive cancer causation. Recent work by Grossart-Maticek[2] and his colleagues in West Germany argues that cancer has no single cause. This is also the finding when looking at cancer using BER techniques. The picture is one of many causes all working together, one of which may be dominant at any time. This is the pattern seen also in chronic illness. The main areas of these causative factors are environmental, psychological and spiritual. The implication is that treatment must be on a similarly broad base, and that no single technique alone will be completely effective. Unfortunately, current approaches to cancer treatment rarely, if ever, ask what has caused the problem. As a result treatment is more or less exclusively directed to getting rid of the 'lump'.

A recent leading article in the *British Medical Journal*[3] looked at environmental causes of cancer. It stated that approximately six million new cases of cancer occur every year in the twenty-four areas of the world for which the United Nations publishes population data. The world-wide number is probably very much higher. It went on to note a striking variation from nation to nation in the patterns of occurrence, which are thought to be due to differences in exposure to environmental risk factors. Even more important is the evidence from migration studies showing that people who move to another country are found to have the pattern of cancers of their new homes within one or two generations (a generation is approximately 27 years). Such studies strongly suggest that as much as 80 to 90 per cent of human cancer is environmentally determined and thus theoretically avoidable. The term 'environmental' embraces all elements of lifestyle — dietary, social, cultural, as well as exposure to carcinogens at work, radiation, drugs etc. The most important environmental cause has been identified as cigarette smoking. As far as diet is concerned, the biggest cancer risks are 'over nutrition', excess fat and meat, insufficient fibre in the diet — in other words, the typical Western diet. Recently, reliable evidence has emerged showing that diets high in fresh fruit and vegetables have a protective effect. This evidence has been further supported by a study which found a deficiency of vitamins A, E and selenium in patients with cancer.

There is a good deal of evidence that psychological causes are important in cancer. A number of studies show that marital stress, such as the death of a spouse or some other event which threatens a persons identity or most important relationship, precedes the diagnosis of cancer by some six to eighteen months. The mechanism of action of these factors is probably mediated through a resulting immune suppression. Psychological profiles of cancer patients have been established by a number of researchers, to the extent that potential cancer victims can be predicted with remarkable accuracy on the basis of personality profiles. The evidence for the reality of environmental and psychological causes comes from standard mainstream medical research. These findings are backed by those of BER readings made on cancer sufferers. Unfortunately, conventional medicine does not apply this research to cancer patients in any effective way as far as treatment is concerned. Alternative therapies in contrast do try to apply these ideas as part of an integrated approach to the problem.

Two further causes have not, as yet, been backed by such solid evidence. One is spiritual causes, which are perhaps difficult to narrow down into a research protocol. The other is the effect of low-level radioactivity. Recently there has been much public disquiet about an apparent increase in the incidence of leukaemias, particularly in children living near to nuclear reprocessing plants. All these observations have been rebuffed by a number of official reports which have looked at the problem from an epidemiological point of view. It is of some interest that these reports have generally failed to quell concern over the environmental risks of long-acting low-level radioactivity, and have generally been perceived as official white-washes. The problem is that from an epidemiological point of view they stand no chance whatever of defining anything but a gross risk, such as that found in cigarette smoking. In other words, the same scientific arguments apply to the study of low-level environmental risks of any sort as to the study of toxicity, or otherwise, of food additives (see Chapter 7). Further developments in BER techniques may possibly help to scientifically define detrimental biological changes occurring as a result of these low-level toxic influences (see Chapter 15).

Cancer Treatment
Conventional treatment approaches are all drastic and centre around surgery, chemotherapy and radiotherapy. Unfortunately the 'gentle approach', in my experience, is not noticeably more effective than the conventional suppressive one so doctors are themselves panicked into using powerful methods to remove the tumour. This is understandable and in some cases can cure, such as in particular leukaemias and certain types of Hodgkin's disease (a cancer of the lymph glands). However, in spite of this, public confidence in mainstream methods of cancer treatment is declining, and if anything this decline is accelerating despite some fairly desperate measures by a number of official cancer research organisations to convince the public that they are finding the answer.

More and more patients are refusing all conventional approaches to their problem, either because they consider them unacceptable or ineffective. Whether these patients fare any worse or better than those who have the appropriate conventional approach is a hotly debated question. This public reaction against conventional approaches to cancer has led to the growth of a number of cancer help centres, largely run by lay staff with some sympathetic medical involvement. There has also been a rapid growth in self-help groups. Together these organizations have adopted a broadly causally-related approach to cancer entirely congruent with Grossart-Maticek's findings, [2] which at best looks at an attempt to treat the psychological, spiritual, nutritional and environmental aspects of the cancer problem. In a few cases the results are impressive but overall, in my view, appear no better than those of conventional medicine, that is as judged by the yardstick of survival.

The alternative cancer movement shows no signs of any attempt to assess their results, and interpret such urgings as pressure from the establishment to expose the 'gentle method' as being bogus. In fact the criteria of success differs fundamentally between the two camps, from the alternative side, includes some factors which are practically impossible to measure (see later). However, the fact that cancer help centres and self-help groups are fulfilling a need is beyond doubt and they are certainly here to stay. It would help if doctors recognized this fact and co-operated with them in a more constructive manner, which would help to minimize the polarization of conventional and alternative approaches.

My own view is that we still lack a truly safe and effective method of fully eradicating a tumour mass. There is the possibility that such a method may be devised, based on some of the ideas which underpin the natural therapies. I am well aware how improbable this suggestion may seem to conventional medical eyes, yet I remain convinced. Only future developments will show whether this hope has any foundation or not.

Nutritional Approaches
These centre around an organic, vegetarian (low fat) diet[4] together with mineral and vitamin supplementation, particularly vitamins A, E and selenium. Sticking to the diet requires great dedication on the part of patients who have grown up with a conventional Western meat-based and junk food diet.

Psychological Approaches

These centre around visualization techniques developed in the 1970s by Carl Simonton,[5] a radiation oncologist, and his wife Stephanie Matthews-Simonton. These methods involve visualizing the body's immune defences acting on the tumour. It is important that the patient's 'thought power' is directed at the healthy tissues around the tumour and not at the diseased cells themselves. Simonton's results are impressive and have been copied worldwide by cancer help centres and self-help groups. The Simonton 'technique' requires great dedication and motivation, just as with the diet, on the part of the patient. The patient-based mutually supportive nature of the cancer help centres and self-help groups is probably a major factor in inducing motivation in even the most hopeless cases, in a way which appears impossible to generate within the relatively formalized rigid structures dominated by nihilistic medical thought as exists in the majority of hospitals today. I have been constantly fascinated by the number of doctors who have developed cancer who have sought my help and have realized how negative and damaging the conventional system is in motivating them and giving them any real hope of recovery. These observations contain many lessons for conventional medicine, lessons which no doubt will be resisted every inch of the way.

Spiritual Approaches

These centre around the various schools of spiritual healers, and those rare psychotherapists and counsellors who are able to identify a spiritual need in the patient, and help him fulfil this need. This is a very difficult area to assess scientifically, but it is hard to dismiss the fundamental changes in those cancer sufferers who are truly able to realize the spiritual meaning of their illness, and then to be able to make the necessary fundamental changes in their lives. This is a sadly neglected approach of conventional cancer treatment, and appears to scare most doctors. The British Holistic Medical Association's motto of 'physician heal thyself' is particularly appropriate in this context.

Complex Homoeopathy

This is able to contribute a great deal in cancer therapy. Not only is it possible to monitor premalignant changes with BER techniques but it is also possible to detect the presence of tiny secondaries, too small to be seen by conventional methods. At the time of writing these claims have not been proven scientifically, but with future developments in BER techniques there is every hope that they soon will be.

The mainstays of complex homoeopathy treatment of cancer is resolving the almost ubiquitous dysbiosis (see Chapter 9), stimulating the liver and pancreas (which are nearly always involved), facilitating lymphatic drainage, and the use of complex homoeopathic degeneration remedies such as *Conium Similiaplexe*, and *Thuja Similiaplexe*. As a rule a complex homoeopathic approach is combined with nutritional, environmental, psychological and spiritual approaches as part of an integrated treatment programme. Complex homoeopathy is a major part of the alternative approach to cancer and should be more widely used together with appropriate BER diagnostic back-up. Unfortunately, however, this concerted attack will not reduce large tumour masses which still require a conventional approach in order to reduce them, of which the least damaging to the body's immune defences is surgery, which is only possible if the tumour is well localized and has not produced multiple secondaries.

Criteria of Success

Most people, and certainly the majority of doctors, take survival time as being the only criteria of success in any cancer therapy. The alternative camp have introduced a new measure, that is, quality of life. This means that the therapeutic approaches which produce appalling side effects (as far as many are concerned) such as complete hair loss, radiation sickness and general debility, score heavily on the negative side when this criterion is taken into consideration. In spite of the manifest reluctance of conventional medicine to attach value to quality of life in all its material, psychological and spiritual aspects, the cultural changes going on in our society, led by the inner directed groups (see Chapter 1) attach more value to quality of life than to its length. This underlines the importance of the sociological changes in society and their relevance to medicine in general and cancer treatment in particular. Conventional medicine ignores this at its peril, and at the continued risk of increasing alienation of patients from the often necessary approaches of conventional medicine.

Conclusion

The cancer debate has only just begun, and it is only recently that there has been an articulate counter to the conventional line, by the burgeoning alternative movement. The alternative approaches are riddled with problems, such as some therapists whose enthusiasm for a particular therapy outweighs their judgement with the result that they practise their particular line with an almost blind omnipotence. A good example is some of the nutritional (dietary) approaches, or some of the spiritual approaches, who by inference claim that diet will cure everything 'because we are what we eat', or because 'the spirit cures all as it is the origin of all'. There is much misdirected reasoning in these statements, and what is needed is an integrated approach with sympathetic non-partisan medical guidance to provide proper judgement, with the result that a truly holistic and potentially maximally effective treatment approach can be devised. This approach is a highly personalized and participatory approach from the patient's point of view, and this in my opinion should be one of the keys to the future of medicine.

14. Holism, a Gathering Force

Holistic medicine means 'whole person' medicine and is something that most doctors claim they practise. In my opinion this is rarely the case.

The medical profession worldwide are suddenly beginning to wake up to the idea of whole person medicine, and this has been marked by the foundaton of the American Holistic Medical Association in 1978, and more recently the British Holistic Medical Association in 1983.

Holism is not just about alternative medicine, but does include these approaches. It is entirely possible to be holistic using conventional therapies alone! In my opinion, however, it is easier if complementary therapies are also used. Claims that alternative therapies are holistic have long been heard, but in fact on their own none of them are. For example, acupuncture is a treatment, not a system of medicine in its own right, and the same applies to homoeopathy. Therefore separately neither can form a truly holistic approach, even though they may well cure a lot of people. This is an important point as it implies that holism is not just about making people well again, it is about the relatedness of all things. The ancient Chinese considered acupuncture to be a system of relationships; therefore in concept it is holistic, but in practice it remains a therapy. The development of this sort of medical system comes as no surprise in a country such as China as the ancient Chinese philosophers considered that the relationships of any object were more important than the object itself. An interesting thought, as in many ways it is much easier to influence something (say a painful elbow) by knowing all its relationships than by knowing everything about the elbow itself in an isolated sense.

In many ways the increasing trend towards holism is a reaction against the dualistic, mechanistic and reductionist base of conventional medicine. It is towards an approach which lends value to the subjective as well as to the objective. In other words things such as loving, caring, touching, hugging, sharing and giving all of a sudden become of real worth in medicine. The fact that they cannot be measured has led to the subjective phenomena being given the 'order of the boot' by conventional scientific medicine. Holistic medicine sees this as misguided and is forcing a re-think at a very basic level as to how we assess whether or not a therapy works.

Principles of Holism
These include the following ideas:

1   Relatedness of all things being of major importance.

2   The concept of balance as succinctly described by traditional Chinese medicine with the Yin/Yang idea, as an indicator of health.

3   Disease being looked upon as an imbalance arising from a faulty relationship or relationships either inside or outside the patient. The key to cure is to identify and correct the relationship.

4   A recognition of the importance of the environment in its material, psychological and social aspects.

5   That any patient is a potentially self-healing system and can be aided on his way by means of therapies which are participatory rather than passive or suppressive.

6   A devolution of power to the patient, with equal power sharing between doctor and patient.

7   A preference for causally directed therapy as opposed to suppressive therapy.

8   An acknowledgement of the spiritual nature of man and a recognition of the validity of subjective experience.

9   A willingness to look at, to use and to assess all the natural therapies and an open-minded yet critical acceptance of the various theories of biological energy.

10 Lastly, but most important of all, a recognition, probably for the first time in modern medicine, that the healer, the physician

himself, should heal himself, as he has been the neglectd part of the healing circuit for far too long.

The Current Biomedical Model

The current biomedical model is dominated by a Newtonian/Cartesian approach to the body. The Cartesian approach comes from the great French philosopher René Descartes who lived nearly 300 years ago. He considered that the human body was a machine: 'Consider the human body as a machine. My thought compares a sick man and an ill-made clock with my idea of a healthy man and a well-made clock'. Descartes affirmed the concept of dualism and helped bring about the separation of body and mind. He was the logical, deductive thinker *par excellence*, and was one of the first to suggest that any phenomenon could be understood by breaking it down into its constituent parts and looking at each part separately. This is the doctrine of scientific reductionism and these ideas underpin the vast majority of modern medical research.

The Future Biomedical Model

The limitations of Descartes' thought have now been recognized by the holistic movement, but there is a worrying tendency for the pendulum to swing too far in the holistic direction. BER techniques show clearly that Descartes was right in part and so indicate that a simultaneous holistic approach is required. The holistic movement hasn't come to this realization yet, and appears to be largely concerned with stress reduction approaches, meditation and psychological approaches. In other words it has adopted a relatively extreme position in the first instance, probably as a reaction against the current biomedical model. Holism will come of age when it incorporates BER medicine and its ideas with its reductionist but also holistic and interrelated approach. I hope that this book will go some way to accelerate this maturation process amongst the holistic movement worldwide.

Physician Heal Thyself

Dr David Zigmond writing in the first *British Journal of Holistic Medicine*[1] has given a masterly account of the doctor's dilemma. Much of this section has been drawn from Dr Zigmond's paper.

He begins by pointing out that doctors have at least double the rate of suicides to the rest of the population. Amongst hospital doctors it is highest amongst psychiatrists who are more likely to commit suicide than their patients, according to some American studies. Doctors make bad husbands and poor fathers and are often workaholic to the detriment of their close personal relationships.

Doctors and others in the caring professions cannot admit the failings which they so readily seek in their patients. The stiff upper lip mentality becomes foremost, particularly in the hospital environment. As a result they develop a false omnipotence. Dr Zigmond then makes the following observation: 'I can only deduce that there is a tacit and severe conspiracy of silence regarding this painful area. Traditionally and still prevalently, the lack of emotional rapport and support within the caring professions is paradoxical but gross'. In other words there is no way out from this rigid situation; much worse, the way medicine is organized exacerbates the situation. The goals set for doctors are career advancement, the attainment of more qualifications, and increasingly hard work. The goals of self discovery and inner development simply don't figure at all and are considered irrelevant by many doctors.

The problem facing doctors, especially, and other members of the caring professions to a lesser extent, is that they are expected to be wise, worldly, patient, strong, unselfish and responsible. They are not expected to be weak, ignorant, indecisive or unable to face the patient's problems. Because the situations a doctor deals with are highly charged, dramatic and in some cases devastating for the patient, the doctor can't take all of this 'on board' and so has to block out many otherwise natural feelings of grief or despair. Doctor Zigmond perceptively points out that this situation leads to 'a kind of emotional anaesthesia or woodenness'. He goes on to say that this leads to a situation where it is impossible to remain a vulnerable, feeling or spontaneous person when subject to years of this kind of demand and control. The effect on intimate relationships is clearly predictable.

The next area Dr Zigmond examines is why doctors need to heal and points out that this can take the form of working out a personal need. When this is stronger than the need to help the patient then the doctor/patient relationship is poisoned and is invariably non-therapeutic from the patient's point of view. Often in this case the doctor will maximize the imbalance of power in the doctor/patient relationship by exaggerating his own status, using amongst other things stage props such as white coats, large desks, lots of minions running around at his beck and call. The patient is expected to be and to remain weak, submissive, and helpless. Hardly a situation in which any participatory approach to healing can be allowed to flourish! Zigmond observes, 'Such dependence upon our patients for our sense of power, self-esteem, worthiness and vicarious expression of locked-up feeling is often not conscious. In the semi-conscious or deeply unconscious mind there are frequently complexes of guilt, and the need for reparation, stemming from our earliest experiences where, in a primitive and irrational manner, we created inordinate notions of the damage we might have done or might still do'. In these situations the doctor who relies on his patients for his sense of power is in fact going through a ritualistic undoing of the feared damage; the problem is that it is an impotent act as it is an incessant undoing. These deep patterns in the psyche of any person working in the caring professions thus needs to be worked out in order to be able to reach anything approaching a truly healing relationship with an equal distribution of power and mutual decision making between doctor and patient.

Zigmond concludes by making the point that the most important way to begin to recognize and deal with these problems is right back at medical school. Medical students ought to be taught in a personally meaningful sense the psychology of the doctor/healer, and the doctors' resultant distress patterns. Those teaching ought to imbue a recognition of the more 'female' intuitive approach, where feelings are given real value. The British Holistic Medical Association itself is a step in the right direction in this area, although in practice the majority of doctors, and medical students as well, remain too armoured and insensitive to accept these lessons at a meaningful personal level.

The Future of Holism

Holism has been tacitly accepted as a valuable idea by the medical profession, as a working ideal it has only been realized by very few indeed. The personal implications of holism are generally resisted, even by many involved in the holistic movement. The importance or otherwise of alternative therapies in holism remains hotly debated, and many feel uncomfortable being involved with therapies they regard as strange and unscientific. Those who have been involved in alternative therapies for some time are justifiably worried that the holistic movement is an attempt by the teaching hospital academic doctors to 'take over' these therapies. Generally speaking the main therapeutic impetus within the British Holistic Medical Association centres around psychological/relaxation approaches with a noticeable neglect of physical therapies and environmental approaches such as clinical ecology. As yet interest has not matured enough to take on board BER medicine. Hopefully as the holistic movement grows it will incorporate the ideas of BER medicine and come to use this approach as a starting point for looking at complicated clinical problems.

Even if the holistic movement is only a doctors' self-help society it will have achieved much.

15. The Medicine of the Future

Much of this book has been about various aspects of a newly emerging system of medicine which looks at the body basically from a point of view of subtle energetic change. I have tried to describe each subject as simply as possible to build up a general picture of the new system of medicine which this book foresees. To that extent all the previous chapters deal with possibilities that exist and are working here and now. To conclude it is necessary to look into the future to examine how things may develop, and to assess the cultural and philosophical implications of the bioenergetic model of man. I wish to record my indebtedness to a friend and colleague Dr Geoffrey Mullarkey for helping me to finally crystallize the ideas of the bioenergetic model of man referred to in this chapter.

The Bioenergetic Paradigm

BER medicine is set firmly within the bioenergetic way of looking at man. However the bioenergetic model owes its origins to the esoteric traditions of a number of ancient cultures, particularly the Chinese and Indian civilizations. It is of major importance for us to understand that the bioenergetic model is therefore culturally foreign to us, and so this makes it very difficult for us to understand it or to experience it in any real sense.

The world of modern experimental science is in tune with our Western culture and is exclusively devoted to the constructs of the five senses. It assumes the separation of the observer from the observed and builds up an image of reality from the information received via the senses. Modern physics is the only area of science which has reached the limit and has forced us to look at the observer (see Chapter 6) and even to consider the role the observer plays in actually creating the reality he perceives. At least that is the implication, but in fact confusion and argument reigns in this area of science.

The bioenergetic view of man regards the relatedness of all things, and of the existence of all things within a single continuum as being what is regarded as reality. Therefore the implication is that the separateness assumed by modern science is not an accurate model of reality. The key factor is that the bioenergetic model describes systems by which we generate the feeling of separateness, and the workings of these systems are all unconscious. Descriptions of these systems and their intricate workings are to be found everywhere in ancient oriental and Ayurvedic texts, they are the workings of the Prana of the Yogis, or the Chi of traditional Chinese medicine. The senses (which by definition are conscious) are one step removed from these subtle energy changes, and by implication from reality. From our cultural point of view this argument is central to the whole issue of any progress in understanding the meaning of subtle energy change in the body. I predict that because of cultural bias the majority of readers will have discarded my argument in this section as being nonsense, as I am suggesting that our senses are one step removed from reality. I would ask those readers to bear with me a little longer.

In order to understand the meaning of subtle energy change we have to do more than simply record that change, we have to build in an understanding of the experiential effects of these changes on the individual and to that extent we cannot exclude the psyche. Therefore a highly individual personalized experience of reality exists. It is likely that BER medicine will develop to recognize the importance of us all experiencing the subtle inner changes in us, which are the bioenergetic flows that govern our workings and perception. This means a long arduous training of 'inward listening', and may well be the future use of meditative states which are now becoming so popular. It may well be that being able to image these subtle changes (see later) may act as a sort of biofeedback system where we could be helped to see the importance of these inner changes and the value of acquiring control over them. Unfortunately current biofeedback is one step removed from this and is firmly rooted in the modern scientific paradigm as it is concerned with the input of the senses exclusively.

If we could learn to be aware of and control these subtle energy changes, rather like some Yogis can do, then we would be well on the way to developing a truly participatory, fundamentally effective, interactive system of health care. This is the key of the bioenergetic message which is ultimately an esoteric one.

Changing Attitudes of the Patient

Currently the majority of patients are not motivated to exercise the laborious self-discipline necessary to develop the inner awareness referred to in the previous section. It is only when we can monitor these changes by visualizing them and seeing their fundamental effect that the majority may begin to see the importance of acquiring control over the body. Those who have followed these meditative techniques have so far been the minority, and have largely done so for intuitive reasons. For the moment the vast majority still prefer the easy way out and use conventional suppressive approaches, rather than face the more arduous and participatory approach of the natural therapies.

Communication between the Paradigms

At the present time the bioenergetic model and the modern scientific view are apparently at loggerheads, and the current 'mind-set' is fundamentally loaded against the bioenergetic model emerging. My own view is that the basic scientific work attempting to monitor and image these subtle energy changes in the body holds the only possibility of changing the situation.

Imaging of subtle electrical change around the body

In the previous section I referred to what I consider to be the most crucial development required in order to bias the current 'mind-set' enough in favour of the bioenergetic model for significant progress to be made. This work centres around visualizing subtle electrical change in the body in the pictorial sense. So far the techniques tried have centred around high voltage high frequency photography (Kirlian Photography).[1] Much of this work has been of a poor scientific standard and has been dogged by artefacts (artificial effects). My own findings in this area have convinced me that all high energy approaches (Kirlian Photography often uses voltage pulses of 20 kilovolts upwards) to monitor subtle energy change are non-starters, as it is not possible to differentiate artefacts from real change in the structures under investigation. My current research direction centres around a number of novel uses of lasers, and so far, in the very early experimental stages, seems to offer a fundamentally better approach to imaging, primarily because it is a low energy approach.

The emerging science of biophysics is consistently finding that very small energy change, for example tiny changes in magnetic fields, are of major biological importance.[2] Recently it has been found that minute electrical potentials co-ordinate the balance of electrical activity in the brain.[3] By comparison a nerve action potential is enormous. Slowly, therefore, evidence is being gathered which leads us to believe that monitoring subtle electrical changes is going to be a useful exercise.

If and when we do ultimately succeed in objectively monitoring these electrical fields will we be able to understand them? My own view is that we will have to use the plethora of incredibly detailed documentation of bioenergetic flow, and influences in the body from oriental and Indian cultures, in order to give some meaning to what we find. Our natural urge to explain and understand these changes will, however, have to be kept in check. I feel that we will have to be content in the first instance with a phenomenological view, rather than rush into too many ill-conceived and limiting explanations of the findings made. I would be very surprised if we reach such a fundamental understanding of these changes in my lifetime, but I certainly expect we will be able to image subtle energy change within the foreseeable future.

Energetic View of Causality

The current bio-medical model looks for single causes; BER medicine shows that a whole spectrum of causes all acting simultaneously, some more dominant than others, is a more accurate view. In other words all illness is a complex outworking of many dynamic influences. From a practical point of view working out the relative importance of each of these influences is crucial in order to be able to determine a truly causally directed treatment regime. As I implied earlier in this chapter, it is highly likely that in future this will involve the patient's psyche in some way.

Conclusion

This chapter is perhaps the most difficult of all to understand, as it touches on many fundamental differences between the bioenergetic and modern scientific model of man. I see and indeed hope for a truly causally orientated, participatory and interactive system of health care developing from the two strands of BER medicine and the emergence of holism. Whether or not this happens depends in many ways on man's spiritual as well as material progress.

Appendix

Addresses of Homoeopathic Pharmacies

Heel Heilmittel Biologische GmbH, D — 7570 Baden-Baden, West Germany.

Dr Madaus & Co., Post Box 910555, 5,000 Koln 91, West Germany.

Pascoe Pharmaceutical Preparations GmbH, 6300 Geissen 1 Schiffenberger Weg 55.
UK Agency — Noma Limited, PO Box 80, Southampton, UK.

Schaper & Drummer, 3320 Salzgitter 61 (Ringelheim), West Germany.

Dr Reckewegg & Co., GmbH, D-6140 Bensheim 1, Berliner Ring 32.
UK Agency — Optimum Health Ltd., 26 Kingston Road, New Malden, Surrey, KT3 3LS.

Wala Heilmittel GmbH, D-7325, Eckwalden, Bad Boll, West Germany.
UK Agency — Weleda, Heanor Road, Ilkeston, Derbyshire.

References

Preface
1 Kenyon J.N., *Modern Techniques of Acupuncture*, Volumes I, II and III. Thorsons, 1983 (Volumes I and II), 1985 (Volume III).

Chapter 1
1 McNulty, C., ' What the Public Want and Think'. A paper given at the 2nd Annual Conference of the British Holistic Medical Association, Oxford, September 1984.
2 Illich, I., *Medical Nemesis* (Boyars, U.K. 1975).
3 Robertson, James, *The Sane Alternative*. Turning Point, The Old Bakehouse, Cholsey, OX10 9NU, U.K., 1983.
4 Handy, Charles, *The Future of Work* (Blackwell, 1984).
5 Capra, Fritjof, *The Turning Point* (Flamingo, 1982).
6 Schwartz, Peter and Ogilvy, J., *The Emergent Paradigm* (Bantam Books, 1985).

Chapter 2
1 Scott, K.A. and McCourt, L.A., *Homoeopathy*, in the 'Alternative Therapists' series (Thorsons, 1982).

Chapter 3
1 Bohm, D. *Wholeness and the Implicate Order* (Routledge & Kegan Paul, 1980).
2 Porkert, M., *Theoretical Foundations of Chinese Medicine: Systems of Correspondence* (MIT Press Cambridge, Mass. USA, 1974).
3 Prigogine, Ilya, and Stengers, I., *Order out of Chaos* (William Heinemann Limited, 1984).

Chapter 4
1 Griggs, B., *Green Pharmacy* (Norman and Hobhouse, 1981) Chapter 20.

2 Hodgkinson, N., *Will to Be Well, the Real Alternative Medicine.* (Hodgkinson, 1984). See also: Hodgkinson, N., 'The bitterest of pills to have to swallow' 'Society Tomorrow', Page 11, *The Guardian,* 6 February 1985.

Chapter 5

1 Kenyon, J.N., *Modern Techniques of Acupuncture* Volume 3 (Thorsons, 1985) Chapter 5. See also: Schimmel, H. edited by Kenyon, J.N., *The Segmental Electrogram* (Vega Grieshaber GmbH & Co., D7622 Schiltach-Schwarzwald, West Germany 1982).

2 Kenyon J.N., *Modern Techniques of Acupuncture* Volume 1, (Thorsons, 1983) Part 2.

3 Kenyon, J.N., *Modern Techniques of Acupuncture* Volume 3. (Thorsons, 1985) Chapter 4.

4 Kenyon, J.N., *Modern Techniques of Acupuncture* Volume 2, (Thorsons, 1983) Chapter 18.

Chapter 6

1 Luthe, W. and Schultz, J.H., *Autogenic Therapy.* (Grune & Stratton, New York, 1969).

2 Shreeve, C. and Shreeve D., *The Healing Power of Hypnotism* (Thorsons, 1984).

3 Minuchin, Salvador, *Families and Family Therapy* (Tavistock Publications, 1974).

4 Rowe, Dorothy, *Depression: The Way Out of Your Prison.* (Routledge and Kegan Paul, 1983).

5 Lawden, D.F., 'Science and Psyche', *Psycho-energetics, the Journal of Psycho-physical Systems.* Vol. 4, No. 4., 387/389, 1982.

6 Einstein, A., Rosen, N., and Podolsky, B., 'Can Quantum mechanical description of reality be considered complete?' *Physics Review,* 47,777, 1935.

7 Hiley, B., 'Quantum mechanics passes the test', *New Scientist,* 17-19, 6 January 1983.

8 Lawden, D.F., 'Separability of Psycho-physical Systems', *Psycho-energetics, the Journal of Psycho-physical Systems,* Vol. 4, No. 1, 1-10 (1981).

9 Lawden, D.F., 'A Berkeleyian model for psychic phenomena'. *Psycho-energies, The Journal of Psycho-physical Systems.* Vol. 5, No. 3, 185/198, 1983.

10 Schmeidler, G.P. and McConnoll, R.A., *ESP and personality patterns* (Yale University Press, 1958).

11 Fisk, G.W. and West, D.J., *Journal of the Society for Psychical Research,* 37, 1-13, 185-197 (1953).

12 Honorton, C., *et al, Journal of the American Society for Psychical Research,* 69, 135 (1975).

13 Taddonio, A., *Journal of Parapsychology* 40, 107, (1976).

Chapter 9

1 Lewith, G.T. and Kenyon, J.N., *Clinical Ecology* (Thorsons, 1985) Chapter 7.

2 Lewith, G.T. and Kenyon, J.N., *Clinical Ecology* (Thorsons, 1985) Chapter 11.

Chapter 13

1 Leading article, *New Scientist,* 8 November 1984, page 2.

2 Grossart-Maticek, R., (a) *Psychotherapy and Psychosomatics* 38. 284-302 (1982) (b) *Psychotherapy and Psychosomatics* 40, 191-210 (1983).

3 Muir, C.S. and Parking, D.M., 'The World Cancer Burden: Prevent or Perish', *British Medical Journal* Vol. 290, pages 5-6, (5 January 1985).

4 Forbes, Alec, *The Bristol Diet* (Century Publishing, 1984).

5 Simonton, Carl O., Matthews-Simonton, Stephanie and Creighton Jones. *Getting Well Again.* (Los Angeles, Tarcher 1978).

Chapter 14

1 Zigmond, David, 'Physician Heal Thyself: the paradox of the wounded healer'. *The British Journal of Holistic Medicine* Vol. I pages 63-71, April 1984.

Chapter 15

1 Dumitrescu, I., Edited by Kenyon, J.N., *Electrographic Imaging in Medicine and Biology.* (Neville Spearman Publishers 1983). Available from C.W. Daniel & Co., 1 Church Path, Saffron Walden, Essex.

2 Kenyon, J.N., *Modern Techniques of Acupuncture* Vol. II. Chapter 18. (Thorsons, 1983).

3 Lerner, E.J., 'Biological effects of electro-magnetic fields, a review paper.' IEEE Spectrum 1984, 57-69.

Index